Healthy Lunchbox

Healthy Lunchbox

The Working Mom's Guide to Keeping You and Your Kids Trim

Rallie McAllister, M.D.

LifeLine
Press®

A Regnery Publishing Company, Washington, D.C.

Library of Congress Cataloging-in-Publication Data available uopn request.

ISBN 0-89526-137-5
Published in the United States by
LifeLine Press
A Regnery Publishing Company
One Massachusetts Avenue, N.W.
Washington, DC 20001

Visit us at www.lifelinepress.com

Distributed to the trade by
National Book Network
4720-A Boston Way
Lanham, MD 20706

Printed on acid-free paper
Manufactured in the United States of America

10 9 8 7 6 5 4 3 2 1

Books are available in quantity for promotional or premium use. Write to
Director of Special Sales, Regnery Publishing, Inc., One Massachusetts
Avenue, N.W., Washington, DC 20001, for information on discounts and
terms or call (202) 216-0600.

This book is dedicated to my three sons,

Chad, who inspires me;

Oakley, who amazes me;

and

Gatlin, who delights me;

and, of course, to my wonderful husband and best friend,

Robin Peavler, M.D., who loves me

Acknowledgments

It takes a village to help an author write a book, and I'd like to thank the people of my village. My deepest gratitude goes to my editor, Molly Mullen, publicist Lauren Lawson, and assistant editor Beth Mottar at LifeLine Press. I will be forever indebted to Michael Ward for going miles out of his way to help me, and to my irrepressible agent, "Mama" Mary Austin, for her bulldog persistence and her heart of pure gold.

For their cheerful assistance with food facts and recipes, I extend warm appreciation to my friends and nutrition specialists Terry Van Huss and Amy Toney. Special thanks to my sister, Gayle Santich, for her listening ear and supportive shoulder, and to my parents, Edward and Maureen Horton, who always encouraged me to take a shot at the moon—as long as my feet stayed on the ground.

Contents

Healthy
Lunchbox

Chapter 1

The Working Mom's Dilemma

If you are the mother of an overweight child, you're by no means alone. You're a kindred spirit to scores of other moms who are growing increasingly concerned about their children's weight. And with good reason. Obesity is currently the most common—and the most serious—medical problem facing our nation's children and possibly your own.

Like adult obesity, childhood obesity is a national epidemic. More than 60 percent of American adults are overweight or obese, up from 45 percent just two decades ago. As this percentage continues to rise, children are following in their parents' heavy footsteps by leaps and bounds, rapidly joining the ranks of overweight adults.

Currently, one of every three kids in the United States has a weight problem, and 11 percent of American children and adolescents are obese. In the past three decades, the number of overweight children of all ages has more than doubled, with most of the increases occurring during the past ten years. Nearly six million kids in the United States now meet the criteria for being overweight or obese.

In general, the term "overweight" refers to children who are 15 percent above their desirable weight, while the term "obese" is used to describe kids who are at least 20 percent over their desirable weight.

Sadly, many overweight kids will grow up to be overweight and obese as adults. While not every overweight child is doomed to a lifelong struggle with weight problems, the risk of remaining obese increases dramatically as children get older. After a child is three years old, the probability that obesity will persist into his adult life rises with each passing year.

Approximately a third of obese preschoolers and half of obese school-aged children will remain obese as adults. By adolescence, overweight kids have a 70 to 80 percent chance of carrying their extra weight into adulthood. Odds like these are incredibly difficult to overcome.

For all its devastating impact on young lives, childhood obesity is only just beginning to be understood. Genetics and cultural influences undoubtedly play an important role. Children of Native American, African-American, and Hispanic heritage are at higher risk for obesity than their Caucasian counterparts. When compared with other parts of the country, the prevalence of childhood obesity in the United States is greater in southern states. Girls are more likely to struggle with their weight than are boys of the same age. Having an overweight parent increases a child's risk of becoming obese, as does belonging to a single-parent home or a low-income family.

Although children meeting these descriptions may have a greater chance of becoming obese, those who don't meet them are by no means immune. The problem of childhood obesity spans both genders, all races, and every economic and educational class.

Maternal Employment: A Mixed Blessing

Why are our children gaining weight at unprecedented rates? One critical factor in the equation of childhood obesity is maternal employment. The rising trend in the percentage of mothers who work outside the home over the last several decades has been closely paralleled by the prevalence of overweight and obese kids. Maternal employment has more than doubled since 1970, a trend mirrored by the rise in childhood obesity during the same time frame.

Studies show a direct, causal relationship between maternal employment and childhood obesity. While the number of weeks worked by mothers over the course of a year seems to exert a minor effect on children's weight status, the total number of hours moms spend at work each week has a significant impact. The more hours a mom works per week, the greater her children's chances of becoming overweight. Sixty-six percent of working mothers clock in forty or more hours per week.

The prevalence of working mothers has skyrocketed in the past century. In 1950, only about 12 percent of American moms worked outside the home. As the women's liberation movement began to gather momentum, women entered the workplace in droves. From 1960 to 1970, the influx of married women workers accounted for almost half the increase in the total U.S. workforce.

With more women trading in their bakeware for briefcases, fewer moms were available for kitchen duty. In the 1940s, moms prepared all of their families' meals from scratch. The advent of frozen food in 1954 opened up a wider—albeit less nutritious—array of food choices to busy women and their families, and the American diet began to change. With mothers having less time to purchase and prepare nutritious meals and snacks, processed foods quickly became dietary staples for both kids and adults.

Around the same time that the TV dinner made its debut, Ray Kroc opened his first franchised McDonald's restaurant, an event that revolutionized American eating habits. The subsequent super-sizing of fast food has undoubtedly contributed to the super sizes of modern-day adults and kids.

By 1987, 57 percent of American mothers were working. Both parents at work meant that even less time was devoted to cooking at home. By the time the eighties rolled around, microwave ovens had become a standard feature in the American home. With the aid of this modern culinary technology, children were now able to fend for themselves in the kitchen, but without the benefit of parental guidance.

By 1998, 74 percent of American women had joined the workforce, and currently, the trend of women working outside the home shows no signs of slacking off. It is projected that by 2005, women will make up nearly half of the nation's total labor force.

With more than two-thirds of U.S. mothers now working for pay, two-earner families are the norm today. A growing number of single women provide most or all of their families' support. As more mothers join the ranks of the gainfully employed, their kids are joining the ranks of the overweight and obese.

The Working Mom Challenge

There are several theories about why children of working moms are more likely to be overweight than those whose mothers stay at home. For starters, mothers who work have greater time constraints than their stay-at-home counterparts. Despite the fact that many moms put in as many hours at work as their husbands or partners, there remains an unequal distribution of labor between men and women when it comes to performing child-related duties and household chores. Women still bear the brunt of the responsibility for the "second shift," which centers primarily on providing food for the children. With less time to shop and prepare meals, working women tend to rely more heavily on fast food and packaged, processed foods to provide nourishment to their families. To complicate matters further, more than a quarter of employed moms work nights or weekends, and more than half work different schedules from their husbands or partners, making sit-down meals at home something of a rarity.

The challenges facing children of working moms start in infancy. More women with infants are working than ever before. Mothers who work may not have the time, flexibility, or energy to breastfeed their newborn babies, or they may stop nursing prematurely in order to return to work after a brief maternity leave. Recent research has highlighted the importance of breastfeeding for the prevention of childhood obesity.

According to the U.S. Bureau of Labor Statistics, the percentage of working moms with children under the age of six has grown dramatically over the past few decades, from 39 percent in 1975 to 64 percent in 2001. This is a critical period in children's lives, when food preferences are being established and cemented. The eating habits developed during the preschool years—whether good or bad—are likely to stick with children throughout their entire lives.

Daycare Drawbacks

Young children of working mothers tend to spend a great deal of their time in daycare centers and other childcare situations, which are often less than ideal. In high-quality childcare arrangements, preschoolers thrive and learn, and older kids are kept safe and supervised after school.

But childcare centers that meet high standards are hard to find for children of any age. Studies show that six out of seven daycare centers provide mediocre to poor-quality care to the children entrusted to them. Ninety percent of family daycare centers, where babies and toddlers spend most of their waking hours, also fall short. At a time when childcare workers typically earn less than animal caretakers, it's little wonder that quality is lacking. Regardless of the quality of the program, there's just no place like home. The daycare environment itself may contribute to childhood obesity, since kids may not be allowed to run as often or play as freely and as actively as they would at home. Low levels of physical activity in the preschool years are closely linked to childhood obesity.

How kids are fed in their early lives has a dramatic impact on their current and future weight status. In childcare situations, kids are typically fed en masse on rather rigid schedules. While moms who keep their toddlers and preschoolers at home are likely to feed their children when they're hungry and willing to eat, daycare workers aren't able to be quite as accommodating. Kids in daycare and preschool programs learn to eat according to the clock, whether or not they're really hungry. As a result, these children may never learn to recognize or rely on their own natural indications of hunger.

While high-quality programs for infants, toddlers, and preschoolers are difficult to find, childcare for older kids may be even scarcer. Only 8 percent of working women have jobs that offer any kind of childcare program, and fewer than 30 percent of public schools offer after-school programs for their students.

Home Alone

Moms may have no choice but to allow their older children to stay at home alone. After school, these kids come home to an empty house and a fully stocked kitchen. Home alone, the latchkey children of working moms fill their long afternoons with junk food and sedentary pursuits. Plugged into televisions, computers, and video stations, these kids typically consume far more calories than they burn.

Kids' afternoon television shows are punctuated regularly with commercial breaks pushing sodas, sugary breakfast cereals, and other junk foods. Slick advertisements bombard kids with seductive messages to eat, eat, and eat some more. With $30 billion spent on the advertisement and promotion of foods and beverages each year, kids are lured to consume diets that are loaded with calories, fat, and sugar and virtually devoid of more beneficial nutrients.

Kids who eat in front of the tube add extra hours to their weekly viewing time, as well as extra inches to their waistlines. Television is strongly linked with childhood obesity; studies show that the more kids watch, the more likely they are to be overweight. Thirty percent of American children currently spend at least five hours a day parked in front of TV sets.

After television, the most popular form of adolescent entertainment is the video game, which involves only slightly more activity than TV viewing. According to one survey of seventh- and eighth-grade students, 60 percent of girls clocked an average of two hours per week playing video games, while 90 percent of boys played for more than four hours a week.

Latchkey kids are more likely to indulge in the mindless inactivity of watching TV and playing video games than kids who spend their afternoons in the company of a parent. Working moms, worried about their children's safety, may not allow their kids to venture outside to play until an adult is at home. Cooped up inside without parental supervision, latchkey kids are left to their own sedentary devices.

Schools: The Latest Health-Free Zone

Working moms need help keeping their kids healthy and active, but they can't count on the public education system to bail them out. If anything, the school system seems to promote childhood obesity. Vending machines purveying high-calorie sodas and snacks are becoming increasingly common fixtures on American middle school and high school campuses. The explosion of candy and soda machines in public schools is a relatively new phenomenon, closely paralleling the rise in childhood obesity. As recently as a decade ago, they were practically nonexistent in public schools.

But as school systems recognized the potential payoff of vending machines, they began signing major contracts with soft drink and snack food companies. In an era of shrinking educational budgets, expanding revenues from soda sales help pay for "extras" like computers and school clubs. According to the National Soft Drink Association, sodas are now sold in at least 60 percent of all public and private middle schools and high schools nationwide. In 1997, kids fed an estimated $750 million into soda and candy vending machines.

Unfortunately, these entrepreneurial school systems are bolstering their budgets at the expense of their students' health and well-being. A recent Harvard study showed a direct link between soft drink consumption and childhood obesity. School kids who regularly consume soft drinks take in approximately 200 more calories each day than their classmates who abstain. While it may not sound like much, an excess intake of even 50 to 100 calories a day can easily lead to a five- to ten-pound weight gain in just one short year.

Soft drinks are a national addiction, with the average American adult now consuming some three hundred cans of the bubbly beverage every year. Grown-ups aren't the only ones who obey their thirst. Kids of all ages are now heavy soft drink consumers, and according to the U.S. Department of Agriculture, they're guzzling sodas at unprecedented rates. Soda consumption among children and adolescents rose roughly 40 percent between 1988 and 1995. In 1979, the typical American teen consumed 20.6 gallons of soda per year, but by 1994, the average teen was downing a whopping 64.5 gallons of soft drinks annually. Kids aged six to eleven are almost as bad, drinking double what their counterparts did twenty years ago. Even preschoolers are official members of the Pepsi generation. Thirty-four percent of American kids aged two to five now drink sodas regularly, and carbonated soft drinks provide more added sugar in a typical toddler's diet than cookies, candy, and ice cream combined.

The dramatic increase in soda consumption is not accidental. Kids are continually pelted with media messages enticing them to drink up. Soft drink manufacturers target their consumers shortly after they emerge from the womb: even baby bottles are branded with product logos. Studies show that kids who regularly drink sodas get shortchanged in several ways. While sodas add little more than empty calories and sugar to children's diets, they also tend to replace more wholesome foods, setting kids up for nutritional deficiencies as well as rapid weight gain.

At the same time that a minefield of vending machines has exploded in U.S. schools, physical activity has become almost an educational after-thought. According to the Centers for Disease Control and Prevention (CDC), fewer than half of American students are currently enrolled in phys-ical education classes.

There is a perfectly logical explanation for the plummeting participation rates. School-based physical education programs have been steadily eroding over the past decade. Just over a third of elementary and secondary schools offer daily physical education classes. High school enrollment in phys ed classes dropped from 42 percent in 1991 to just 25 percent in 1995.

Not only are fewer classes available, but also the class period has been shortened, and kids aren't required to exercise as vigorously as they were in the past. Without regular or effective physical education periods, kids may have few opportunities to sweat off extra calories. More important, they don't learn to exercise properly and may never become involved in fit-ness programs throughout their entire lives.

Junk Food

Lack of exercise combined with an ever-increasing consumption of junk foods piles additional pounds on kids. Because junk foods don't belong in any one of the five major food groups, they have limited nutritional value. Kids whose diets are rich in junk food get loads of salt, sugar, fat, and calo-ries, but little in the way of vitamins and minerals.

According to a recent study in the *American Journal of Clinical Nutrition*, one-third of the typical American diet is made up of junk food. The average American gets 27 percent of total daily energy from junk foods, and nearly a third of Americans consume nearly half of their daily calories in the form of these non-nutritious foods.

Nine out of ten products that food manufacturers hawk to children meet the criteria for junk food. Packaged in alluring cartoon wrappers, with "free" toys, prizes, and games inside, they're practically impossible for kids to resist. In addition to being high in calories and fat, these foods take the place of more nutritious ones, leaving kids at risk for deficiencies of important vitamins, minerals, and other nutrients.

Recognizing the dual problems of increasing accessibility to non-nutritious foods and childhood obesity, Uncle Sam decided to get more involved. In 1990, the U.S. Food and Drug Administration replaced the more familiar "four food groups" with the Food Guide Pyramid (see p. 68), encouraging American adults and kids to reduce the fat in their diets. In 1993, new food labels providing comprehensive nutrition information were introduced in an effort to give Americans more control over their dietary intake.

Incredibly, only 1 percent of U.S. children and adolescents currently consume a diet that meets the recommendations of the Food Guide Pyramid. Numerous studies have verified that kids who consume less than ideal diets are more likely to have behavioral and academic problems than those who are properly nourished.

The very act of living in the United States puts every American man, woman, and child at risk for obesity. Becoming overweight in childhood seems to be a normal response to the American culture, and remaining thin in our food-focused society requires almost a superhuman effort.

Health Problems and Obesity

Regardless of the causes of childhood and adult obesity, our growing waistlines come with a growing price tag to the nation. Obesity-related illnesses cost Americans nearly $130 billion each year. People who become overweight in adulthood typically start experiencing obesity-related health problems around the ripe old age of fifty. But with children starting out as obese adults, they're beginning to experience weight-related disorders and diseases prematurely—often as early as their twenties. Although some mothers work hard to convince themselves that childhood obesity is largely a cosmetic problem, the real consequences are far graver. Tragically, six million kids nationwide are so overweight that their health is in danger. For the first time in a century, American kids face a shorter life expectancy than their parents.

Heart Disease

Heart disease is currently the number-one killer of U.S. adults. According to the CDC, nearly 60 percent of overweight kids between the ages of five and ten already have at least one of the risk factors for heart disease, which include high blood pressure and elevated levels of blood sugar and insulin. Twenty percent of young Americans have high cholesterol levels, and boys as young as fifteen are developing clogged arteries.

The onset of these risk factors in childhood results in both immediate and long-term damage to the cardiovascular system. Atherosclerosis, commonly known as hardening of the arteries, has its origins in childhood. Diets rich in cholesterol and fat, like the typical American fare, lead to the buildup of plaques on artery walls. When these plaques form on the blood vessels of the heart, they dramatically increase the risk of heart disease.

The risk of future heart disease is so great among young people that the American Heart Association recently published guidelines for cardiovascular health for children, recommending the same sort of lifestyle measures that are standard for adults. Cardiologists are advising kids to refrain from smoking, eat a well-balanced, nutritious diet that is low in fat and cholesterol, and get plenty of regular exercise.

It might seem that these words of wisdom would be unnecessary for children, but the earlier preventive behaviors are started, the better off children will be. With 33 percent of kids overweight, 20 percent of high school seniors smoking, and fewer than 25 percent getting regular exercise, kids of all ages are setting the table for heart disease in early adulthood. America's youth are in grave danger of developing—and dying of—heart disease at a much younger age than folks of their parents' generation.

Cancer

Heart disease is just one serious consequence of childhood overeating and obesity, and unfortunately, there are many others. A recent study suggests that children who overeat may have a greater risk for developing certain types of cancer in adulthood. Higher levels of food intake are linked to cancers of the breast, colon, and pancreas, among others.

For each 250-calorie increase in a child's daily diet, the risk of developing certain cancers rises by approximately 20 percent. These findings confirm the importance of establishing good nutritional habits early in childhood. They also suggest that the unfavorable trends seen in the increase of some cancers may have their origins early in life.

Type II Diabetes

Over the last two decades, a new and frightening public health problem has emerged in the United States: Type II diabetes is appearing in unprecedented rates among children and adolescents. Like pediatric obesity, type II diabetes in children has become surprisingly common. Currently, 25 percent of obese American children are showing early signs of the disease.

Ten years ago, no one could have imagined that type II diabetes would strike children at the present rate. In the not too distant past, this type of diabetes was so rarely seen in children that its official moniker was "adult-onset" diabetes. That's no longer the case, according to the American Diabetes Association. The percentage of children with newly diagnosed diabetes who are classified as having type II diabetes has risen from less than 5 percent before 1994 to nearly 50 percent in subsequent years.

Among U.S. children, the average age at diagnosis of type II diabetes is between twelve and fourteen, corresponding with the onset of puberty. The disease affects girls more often than boys, and children of non-European origin are at greatest risk for developing the disease. Type II diabetes is strongly linked to poor eating habits, sedentary lifestyles, and a family history of diabetes. While these factors all play important roles in the development of type II diabetes in childhood, there is little doubt that the primary instigator of the disease is excess body weight.

Type II diabetes is typically a lifelong disease that develops when the body becomes resistant to insulin, usually as a result of being overweight or obese. Insulin, a hormone produced by the pancreas, helps the body use sugar from the diet by transporting it to the cells in body tissues. Insulin resistance is characterized by the inability of fat, muscle, and liver cells to use insulin properly. As more and more insulin is needed to transport sugar in the body, the insulin-producing cells of the pancreas begin to falter, unable to keep up with the increasing demand for the hormone. As a result, sugar begins to accumulate in the bloodstream, leading to type II diabetes.

Weight loss in some overweight children and adults with early signs of type II diabetes can occasionally be curative. In its initial stages, the disease can sometimes be managed with a strict diet and exercise program, but with time, most people will require pills or insulin injections to keep their blood sugar levels under control.

Over time, elevated blood sugar levels can damage nerves, organs, and blood vessels throughout the body. The longer a person has diabetes, the greater his chances of developing the disabling or life-threatening consequences of the disease. These consequences include blindness, kidney failure, heart attacks, strokes, and infections that require foot and leg amputations.

In the past, the complications associated with type II diabetes were seen primarily in older adults in the fifth and sixth decades of their lives. The development of type II diabetes in childhood forebodes serious health problems in adulthood. Diabetic youngsters will begin to suffer complications much sooner in life, and the consequences will undoubtedly be deadly.

Type II diabetes among children and adolescents is, for the most part, a preventable disease. By helping kids to eat nutritious, well-balanced diets, exercise regularly, and avoid excessive weight gain, moms can help safeguard their kids against this devastating disease.

Bone Fractures and Osteoporosis

Recent studies have demonstrated that overweight and obese kids are at greater risk for bone fractures in childhood and the development of osteoporosis in adulthood. Several factors are thought to be responsible for this phenomenon. Overweight children are less likely to have been breastfed in infancy, and some of the milk substitutes commonly used in commercial infant formula lack important nutrients that promote optimal bone health.

Many overweight children spend most of their days indoors, parked in front of television sets and plugged into computer screens. Because these activities limit the time spent outside, kids may not get enough exposure to sunlight. Lack of sunlight can result in deficiencies in vitamin D, a substance necessary for the growth and development of strong bones.

Overweight children are more likely to consume less nutritious foods and beverages than their normal-weight counterparts. Diets that are lacking in calcium contribute to weaker bones. Consumption of soft drinks provides kids with excess caffeine, sodium, and phosphorus, and these substances are known to interfere with calcium absorption by the body.

Physical activity in children is a strong predictor of bone thickness and bone strength in both children and adults. Since overweight kids are less likely to exercise regularly than normal-weight children, they end up with thinner, weaker bones than their more active counterparts.

Respiratory Diseases

Obese children are at risk for developing a slew of respiratory diseases, including asthma and obstructive sleep apnea. Approximately 30 percent of obese children in the U.S. have been diagnosed with asthma, compared with 5 to 12 percent of the general population.

Obesity is commonly associated with sleep apnea in kids. Excess weight gain can result in the deposition of extra fatty tissue in the neck and mouth, making it more difficult for overweight children to breathe properly while they sleep. As a result, kids with obstructive sleep apnea may be partially awakened dozens to hundreds of times each night, as they gasp for air and struggle to reopen their airways. Because kids with obstructive sleep apnea aren't able to get a good night's rest, they're often tired and grumpy during the daytime. Several studies have found that kids with sleep apnea perform poorly in school. Their fatigue often interferes with their ability to pay attention, and they may end up being erroneously diagnosed with attention deficit disorder or other learning disabilities. In overweight kids with obstructive sleep apnea, weight loss is almost always curative.

Psychological Consequences

While the physical problems associated with excess weight are bad enough, the emotional and psychological damage resulting from childhood obesity can be even worse.

Many of the physical complications of obesity may not be manifested until adulthood, but the psychological consequences of the condition begin very early in life. In America's fat-phobic culture, obesity bears a huge negative social stigma. Overweight children are subjected to teasing and ridicule more often than kids without weight problems. At a time in life when egos are already extremely fragile and vulnerable, enduring this type of humiliation can be emotionally devastating.

Overweight children report enduring traumatic and stigmatizing experiences, including name-calling and cruel comments from family members, friends, and even total strangers. It's little wonder that these kids have higher rates of anxiety and depression and attempt suicide more frequently than children without weight problems.

Obese children have been shown to suffer from low levels of self-esteem, which in turn can make them more likely to drink alcohol, smoke cigarettes, and engage in risky sexual behaviors than kids who feel better about themselves. When compared with their normal-weight peers, overweight kids have a greater tendency to suffer from sadness, loneliness, and feelings of isolation. They exhibit a greater sense of rejection and failure and tend to have poor interpersonal skills. Self-consciousness and shame about their bodies interfere with their ability to develop social interests and become part of fulfilling relationships. Sadly, their excess weight—along with the social stigma it carries and the pain it inflicts—will follow most obese children into adulthood.

If you have a child who is overweight, it's not too late to turn things around. Helping your child lose weight and keep it off may be one of the most challenging tasks that you face as a mother. But if you don't step forward and accept that challenge, who will? When you help your child lose weight, you'll be giving him the foundation he needs to enjoy a lifetime of good health and happiness.

Chapter 2

The Mom Connection

Of all the people in your children's world, you have the most powerful influence on their eating behaviors. This influence is established very early in life, starting on day one of existence, when you feed your newborn baby his or her very first meal.

Maternal nurturing behaviors are deeply rooted in the act of feeding. Providing nutrition to children is one of the most important and emotionally rewarding parts of motherhood. As a rule, moms are deeply gratified when they offer love to their infants in the form of formula or breast milk, and they feel that their love is returned when the child accepts the gift of food by partaking of it.

On the other hand, while children may not consciously remember, their earliest sensations of fulfillment and satisfaction come from the process of being held, comforted, and fed. When mothers and infants engage in the mutual act of feeding, it's a time of intense bonding. Mother and child meld their bodies together, gaze lovingly into each other's eyes, and share special smiles as the child nurses from the breast or bottle. These early feeding experiences shape children's eating behaviors for the rest of their lives.

Mom: The Nutritional Gatekeeper

From the beginning of time, mothers have been charged with safeguarding their families' nutritional health. Although more moms are working outside the home than ever before, their traditional role has changed very little.

With the hectic pace of modern life, increasing time constraints are making it tougher for working moms to meet the demands of their role as the nutritional gatekeepers for their families. After a long, exhausting day at work, many women may feel they simply don't have the time or the energy to prepare delicious, nutritious meals or to supervise their children's eating and exercising behaviors. Nonetheless, mothers have a unique opportunity—and a responsibility—to teach their children about the benefits of sound nutrition and a healthy lifestyle.

Before mothers can educate their children, they must first educate themselves. A recent U.S. Department of Agriculture study found that the more a mother knows about nutrition, the less likely her children are to be overweight.

Maternal Obesity

As the old saying goes, the apple doesn't fall far from the tree. When it comes to predicting whether or not a child will be overweight or obese as an adult, you don't have to look much farther than his mother. Maternal obesity or overweight is the single most important predictor of obesity in children.

Children of overweight moms are dramatically more likely to be overweight themselves than children of normal-weight moms. This pattern exists even when kids are reared apart from their biological mothers, indicating a strong genetic contribution.

While heredity is undoubtedly a critical factor, it doesn't necessarily doom a child to a lifetime of obesity. The home environment in which a child is raised seems to be equally as important as his genes. In fact, the genetic predisposition to gain weight is expressed only when children are reared in surroundings that are conducive to weight gain. While genetics may load the gun, the environment seems to pull the trigger.

Fortunately, although moms make a major contribution to the genetic makeup of their children, they're also in charge of creating the home environments in which their kids are raised. What moms are lacking in terms of genetics gifts, they can make up in other ways.

Although a mother's weight status has the greatest impact on her children's risk of becoming overweight or obese, the influence of the father cannot be ignored. Children with one obese parent have a 40 percent chance of becoming overweight or obese themselves. In families where both parents are obese, nearly 80 percent of children will develop the condition. On the other hand, only 7 percent of children with two parents of normal weight become obese.

Physical Activity

Mothers' levels of physical activity are also strongly correlated with their children's weight. Sedentary mothers are likely to have equally sluggish offspring, and this lack of exercise is closely linked to weight-control problems. The good news is that the opposite is also true: Children of active parents are roughly six times more likely to be physically active than kids whose parents are couch potatoes.

Dieting Moms

Although overweight and sedentary moms are more likely to have obese children than their lighter, more active maternal counterparts, even thin moms aren't perfect. Thin mothers who maintain their girlish figures with rigorous dieting, poor food choices, and unhealthy exercising behaviors send dangerous messages about food and eating to their highly suggestible children.

Although it may seem perfectly logical that moms who are highly weight-conscious would have thin, healthy kids, the opposite is actually true. Maternal food fears, fixations, and phobias exert a profound negative influence on children. Moms who are obsessed with the minute-to-minute fluctuations in their weight and who fret out loud about every gram of fat

(continued on page 20)

Mom's Middle-Age Spread

It's just another one of life's precious little milestones, like walking, losing
your first tooth, or finding the acne equivalent of Mount St. Helen's erupting
from your formerly clear complexion. Sometime around the age of forty,
your body undergoes yet another metamorphosis, and you begin what is
known as the middle-age spread.

For most women, the addition of a new pair of love handles isn't exactly a
cause for celebration, but it seems that we are doomed to spread with age.
Currently, half of all Americans over the age of fifty are overweight. As we
grow older, we tend to pack on extra pounds, and what's worse, those
pounds tend to pile up in all the wrong places, like in the double-chin section or the spare-tire department.

When it comes to your health, fat stored in the midsection of the body is
the most dangerous kind. This type of fat, called visceral fat, wedges itself
around your intestines and the vital organs of your chest and abdomen.
Abdominal fat is not only unsightly, it's also most closely linked to the health
risks of obesity.

Doctors unceremoniously group their patients into one of two categories,
depending on their patterns of weight distribution. Women who store most
of their body fat around their midsections are referred to as "apples," while
women who deposit more fat around their hips and thighs are considered to
be "pears."

Thanks to the influence of the female hormone estrogen, most premeno-
pausal women are pears. While this body type is a significant source of cos-
metic concern for most of us girls, we can take comfort in the knowledge
that it doesn't pose a major health risk. After menopause, waning estrogen
levels cause women to adopt a more masculine pattern of fat distribution. As
fat deposits in the midsection expand, these women join the ranks of the
apples.

You probably already have a good idea which fruit you most resemble. If
you're not sure, you can take the acid test and stand naked before a full-

length mirror (don't forget to turn the lights on). You may be pleasantly surprised to find that your body doesn't resemble either an apple or a pear, but rather a green bean.

If you fear that your eyes might deceive you, there's an easy way to find out which fruit you most resemble in the privacy of your home. You can determine your waist-to-hip ratio simply by measuring your waist at its narrowest point, your hips at their widest point, and then dividing the waist measurement by the hip measurement. A waist-to-hip ratio greater than 0.8 for women is indicative of an apple shape.

Although avoiding the middle-age spread is one of life's great challenges, you shouldn't accept it without a good fight. Even weight gains as small as ten extra pounds and increases of just two extra inches around your middle can jeopardize your health. Over thirty-nine chronic illnesses are linked to these types of expansions, including type II diabetes, high cholesterol levels, and hypertension. Excess abdominal fat increases the risk for heart disease, gout, osteoarthritis, and cancers of the breast, colon, and uterus.

Staying physically fit as you grow older takes a great deal more effort than it did when you were a mere spring chick. Starting around your thirtieth birthday, your metabolic rate drops by about 1 percent each year. As a mature adult, you'll need to eat somewhere between 200 and 400 fewer calories each day than you did in your youth if you want to maintain your weight. If you don't fine-tune your eating habits or devote more time to exercise, you can expect to gain about three to five pounds each and every decade after the grand old age of thirty-five.

If you've already begun the amoeboid-like spread of middle age, don't despair. The good news is that you don't have to achieve your high school graduation weight to be healthy. A loss of just 10 percent of your current weight has dramatic benefits, significantly lowering your risk for most obesity-related diseases. If the middle-age spread is a milestone that you'd rather not achieve, a little extra effort in the diet and exercise department can go a long way toward postponing it. If you work really hard, you may be able to prevent it altogether.

or cholesterol they consume actually contribute to the problem of child-hood obesity, not to mention growth and developmental abnormalities. Even worse, they tend to deepen kids' natural insecurities about their own developing and rapidly changing bodies.

The dieting practices of moms have a tremendous influence on their children's emerging ideas and beliefs about nutrition and weight status, even at the tender age of five years. Moms who are constantly bemoaning their weight and chronically dieting have the greatest negative impact on their daughters, rather than their sons. This may help explain why an estimated 80 percent of all ten-year-old girls are terrified of being fat.

Maternal Influence on Eating Behaviors

During their early years, children are busy forming attitudes about foods and developing the eating habits—good or bad—that will follow them throughout their lives. Food preferences are firmly established as early as five years of age. For this reason, the first five years of children's lives are critical in terms of providing them with an understanding of what consti-tutes a well-balanced diet. It's also the best time to introduce them to a wide variety of nutritious foods that they can continue to eat and enjoy as they grow older. But perhaps even more important than how a mom manages her child's diet is how she manages her own. Children model their own eating behaviors after both of their parents, but especially their mothers.

As the most influential person in her child's life, a mother sets the stage for childhood eating behaviors. Whether they realize it or not, moms are constantly in the spotlight, providing their children with a steady stream of information about when, what, and how much to eat.

Kids are quick to pick up and mimic the environmental cues that trigger eating in the adults around them, especially their moms. As kids continue to grow and develop, these cues become deeply engrained and cemented. Eventually, children learn to respond to the same eating cues as their mothers, without giving them much conscious thought.

If a child sees Mom use food for comfort, to relieve stress, or as an escape from boredom, chances are great that the child will turn to food for the same reasons. If a mother shows lack of restraint when eating, her children are likely to do the same. The more a child uses food for non-nutritive purposes, and the less restraint he exerts over his eating behaviors, the more likely he is to be overweight, both in childhood and as an adult.

As the primary role model in your child's life, you must lead by your own positive example. You must choose nutritious foods to eat, avoid excessive snacking, and try to limit your own food intake to appropriate amounts.

Overly Restrictive Moms Versus Overly Permissive Moms

Fostering the establishment of healthy eating patterns in youngsters requires a variety of mothering skills that improve not only the health of children but their overall well-being. This maternal bag of tricks includes the ability to set limits, establish consistent but flexible routines, and anticipate children's needs. Moms must be able to maintain physical and emotional closeness with their children and learn to read their kids' nonverbal cues. Above all, moms must continually teach, encourage, and model desirable behaviors. Developing these parenting skills—and then sticking with them—can be a challenge for any mother.

When it comes to overseeing a child's diet, moms must walk a very thin line. Mothers who allow their children too much freedom of choice in terms of selection, timing, and quantities of food eaten are setting their children up for a lifetime struggle with weight issues. On the other hand, mothers who aggressively restrict their children's diets are just as bad. Both the overly permissive mother and the overly restrictive mother are more likely to have overweight and obese children than moms who consistently provide nutritious foods for their children in a relaxed, nonjudgmental manner.

Who's in Charge?

If you're concerned that your child is overweight, and you want to help her slim down, it seems only natural that you should carefully structure her eating habits and restrict her food intake. But as it turns out, these approaches can actually be more harmful than helpful. An increasing body of scientific literature suggests that a child's risk of becoming or remaining obese is dramatically increased when her mother exerts a high degree of control over her eating behaviors.

When mothers take it upon themselves to monitor every morsel of food their children eat, the results are devastating. Children quickly lose the ability to regulate their own appetites. They learn to eat in response to external cues (their mothers' wishes) rather than rely on their own internal cues (hunger and satiety).

Examples of excessive maternal control include insisting that children eat only at certain times or that they eat everything that is served to them. Children who are forced to eat according to rigid schedules often end up eating when they're not really hungry. Forcing kids to "clean" their plates may push them to eat more food than they want or need.

In order to obey Mom, these kids have to ignore their bodies' messages that they are full. If children are continually forced to override their own internal satiety signals, they will eventually lose touch with them. As a result, they no longer have the ability to regulate their own food intake properly.

It has also been shown that using food as a reward leads to childhood overeating and obesity. Mothers who resort to this type of control tactic have a profound negative influence on their kids' food preferences. Children learn to dislike certain foods, like green vegetables, when they are required to eat them in order to obtain rewards, like desserts. While kids are under the watchful eye of their mothers, they may choke down the "bad" food (green beans) in order to obtain the reward of a "good" food (chocolate cake). But as soon as they're out from under Mom's controlling thumb, they'll simply bypass the green beans and make a beeline for the cake.

The use of food as a reward is a surefire way to instill bad eating habits in your kids, and it sends your child mixed messages about food. It doesn't make much sense to treat your child to an ice cream cone as a reward for sticking with an eating or exercise program.

While moms should encourage their children to select foods that support a healthy and well-balanced diet, they shouldn't demand that their kids eat certain foods. You can increase your child's willingness to try new foods by asking him just to *taste* the new food, rather than insist that he *eat* it. If you give your child the option of just licking a new food with his tongue, he'll be more likely to try it. Assure him that if he takes a bite and decides he doesn't like it, he'll be allowed to spit it into a napkin.

When you promote the introduction of new foods in a positive manner, it allows control of eating behaviors to remain where it belongs—with your child. At the same time, it gives him the freedom and the courage to experiment with new foods.

You can foster your children's preferences for nutritious foods and promote their acceptance of new foods without resorting to negative actions, like labeling foods as "good" or "bad," making certain foods off limits, or pressuring kids to eat. No matter how good your intentions might be, you must avoid becoming a food cop. Instead, you must strive to make every eating experience a relaxed and positive affair.

One of the greatest gifts you can give your children is the freedom to respond to their internal signals of hunger and satiety. Allow them to regulate their own food intake. Your responsibility as a mother is to make a variety of tasty, nutritious foods available to your children for meals and snacks. Decisions about which of those foods to eat, how much to eat, or whether to eat anything at all belong entirely to the child.

Recognizing Obesity in Your Child

Obesity tends to be in the eye of the beholder, and many parents are incredibly reluctant to behold their children as overweight. One study revealed that among mothers and fathers whose children clearly met the criteria for obesity, 35 percent of those parents did not perceive their children as having a weight problem at all.

Reluctance to label children as "overweight" or "obese" may stem from cultural beliefs about body size. Some ethnic groups view children and adults with larger physiques as being healthier, stronger, and more attractive than their thinner counterparts. But for many parents, the failure to recognize overweight or obesity in their own children has nothing at all to do with cultural influences; it is simply a matter of denial.

Denial is very common in both fathers and mothers of obese children. Some may try to convince themselves that their child's extra weight is due to "big bones" or a "healthy appetite." Parents frequently rationalize their children's weight problems, saying that they aren't really overweight, but rather have a lot of "baby fat" and will eventually outgrow it.

Many mothers make the subconscious decision to overlook or ignore their children's weight problems because they feel guilty. They may feel that they're the ones to blame for their children's poor eating habits. If moms are overweight themselves, they may feel helpless or hypocritical about addressing weight problems in their children.

Some moms believe that since everyone else in the family has a weight problem, their children are simply genetically doomed to be overweight. They may be reluctant to involve themselves or their children in what may seem to be a futile struggle against destiny.

Among other mothers, there is a certain amount of fear that drawing attention to their children's weight will backfire, leading to eating disorders or dangerous dieting practices. If this is the case, you can take comfort in the knowledge that while 33 percent of children are overweight or obese, anorexia affects only about one in two hundred children between the ages of twelve and eighteen, with most of them being girls.

It's not uncommon for moms to avoid addressing a child's weight problem because they feel powerless to change it. Many lament that they have no control over their children's eating or exercising behaviors. These are the moms who say things like, "Joey just refuses to exercise. He'd rather play video games," or, "I can't get Abby to eat vegetables or drink milk. She only wants french fries and soft drinks."

Contrary to popular belief, there is no scientific evidence to support the notion that kids have an innate, unlearned, preprogrammed preference for foods that are high in fat or calories. What is true is that parents tend to keep foods that they like in their homes, and they tend to eat them in front of their children. Following the bad examples set by their mothers and fathers, children naturally include many of their parents' favorite foods in their own diets and are likely to develop preferences for high-fat foods.

The best way to get kids to eat nutritious foods in a noncontrolling, hands-off manner is to stock your kitchen with only those foods that you want your children to eat. If you don't want your kids eating potato chips, don't bring them home from the store.

Childhood obesity is an extremely delicate issue that is fraught with emotional tension, and it must be addressed in sensitive, positive ways. Before it can be addressed, it must first be recognized and accepted by mothers and their children. What moms believe about their children's condition of overweight has a strong impact on the nutritional practices and exercise activities they implement and enforce.

How do you know if your child is overweight in the first place? Since mothers are notoriously poor at judging their own children's weight status, it's important to enlist your pediatrician's help. In general, the term "overweight" refers to children who are 15 percent above their desirable weight, while the term "obese" is used to describe kids who are at least 20 percent over their desirable weight. If the pediatrician determines that your child is overweight or obese, she may be able to make some suggestions about helping your child slim down. The doctor will also be able to determine if your child's weight problem is due to a medical condition, which, although unlikely, is still a possibility that needs to be ruled out.

Body Mass Index

As part of a routine examination, your child's height and weight will be measured. Starting when your child is two years old, pediatricians usually begin plotting these measurements on a specialized graph to assess his weight status. The charts that doctors use are the Body Mass Index percentile growth charts, developed by the CDC. These charts are age-specific, and they compare your child's measurements with those of children who are the same age. Separate charts are used for boys and girls to account for the differences in growth rates and percentages of body fat present as the two genders mature. The data are recorded in your child's medical record, and over time, the pattern established by the plotting of periodic measurements allows your pediatrician to track your child's growth and weight gain.

The charts are based on a measurement called the Body Mass Index, or BMI. Although BMI is not a direct or perfect measure of body fat, it correlates fairly reliably, making it reasonably accurate. Because of its reliability and ease of use, the BMI has become a standard tool used to identify kids that are overweight and obese. Obesity, defined as an excess accumulation of body fat, is present when total body weight is more than 25 percent fat in boys and more than 32 percent fat in girls.

BMI is calculated by dividing a child's weight in kilograms by his height in meters squared. Children with a BMI that falls between 25 and 29.9 are considered to be overweight. A BMI in this range corresponds to a weight that puts a child at greater than 85th percentile, meaning that your child weighs more than 85 percent of children of the same height, age, and gender.

If a child's BMI is 30 or greater, he is considered to be obese. A BMI of 30 corresponds to a weight that falls at or above the 95th percentile, meaning that the child weighs more than 95 percent of other children of the same age, gender, and height. In general, if a child's weight is between 20 and 30 percent in excess of the expected weight for a given height, he is considered to be mildly obese. If his weight is 30 percent or more above the desirable body weight, he is considered to be severely obese.

The BMI percentile charts on the following pages will allow you to familiarize yourself with the tools and get a general idea of where your child currently stands.

It's not a good idea to follow your poor kid around with a scale and a tape measure to see how he stacks up on a daily basis. Only those measurements taken in the pediatrician's office should be plotted on the chart. Measurements taken at home tend to be a little less than accurate, and because of the manner in which the BMI is determined, even small measuring mistakes can result in big errors in BMI calculations.

When you try to decipher BMI readings for your child, it is important to look at them as a *trend* instead of worrying about individual numbers. Any one measurement taken alone or out of context might give you a skewed impression about your child's weight status. Since individual BMI measurements normally fluctuate with age and throughout the growth process in children, the real value of the BMI lies in its ability to establish a pattern over time.

This pattern allows both doctors and moms to watch children's growth and weight gain and determine whether they are normal compared with those of children of the same age and gender. If your child's BMI is fol-

BMI for Boys

Body Mass Index-for-age percentiles for boys 2 to 20

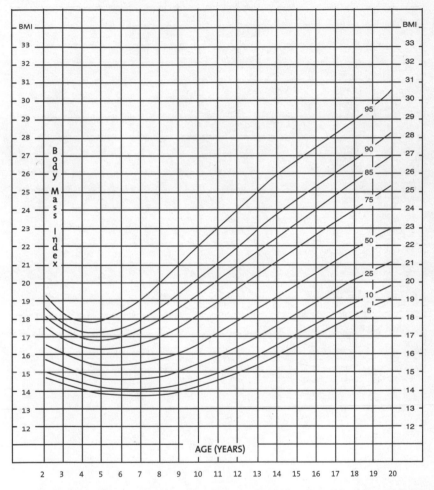

SOURCE: Developed by the National Center for Health Statistics in collaboration with the National Center for Chronic Disease Prevention and Health Promotion (2000).http://www.odc.gov.growthcharts

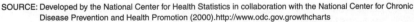

lowing a rising trend, it gives you a chance to take action before he becomes seriously overweight or obese.

Adults can also use BMI charts to determine whether they are overweight or obese. For adults, the optimal BMI for good health is thought to

BMI for Girls

Body Mass Index-for-age percentiles for girls 2 to 20

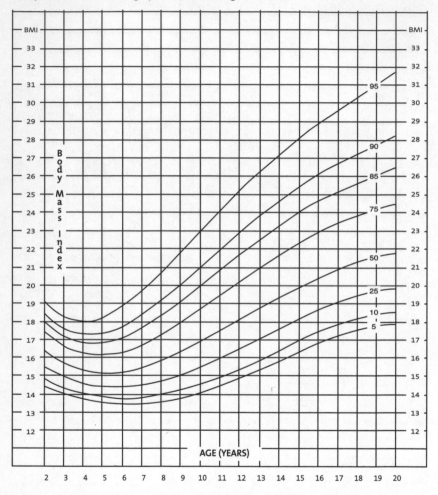

SOURCE: Developed by the National Center for Health Statistics in collaboration with the National Center for Chronic Disease Prevention and Health Promotion (2000).http://www.odc.gov.growthcharts

be in the range of 19 to 21 for women and 20 to 22 for men. If your BMI is a little higher, don't worry. Anyone with a BMI of 18.5 to 24.9 is still considered to be of normal weight. But if you currently have a BMI of 25 to 29.9, you're considered to be overweight.

Obesity itself is divided into three classes. A BMI of 30 to 34.9 puts you in obesity class I; while a BMI of 35 to 39.9 puts you in obesity class II. People with BMIs of 40 or above are considered to be extremely obese, and they fall into obesity class III. If you find yourself in one of these categories, it's time to get to work.

Obesity aside, you can use the BMI to assess your overall health. In general, a BMI that is 24 or less is consistent with good health, while a BMI of 27 or greater is associated with a greater risk of type II diabetes, heart disease and stroke, degenerative joint diseases, and many types of cancer.

It's time to find out exactly where you stand by using the BMI chart for adults on the next page.

Psychological Consequences of Obesity

Regardless of how willing mothers are to ignore or rationalize their children's excess weight, kids' peer groups are not so forgiving. Overweight and obese children suffer terribly in terms of emotional pain, and their mothers may not have any idea about the embarrassment or humiliation that their kids are experiencing. Many overweight kids don't tell their moms about the torment they endure. Some kids feel ashamed and embarrassed, and talking about it is just too painful for them.

But even when kids say nothing, they're undoubtedly getting the "fat is bad" message, loud and clear. In spite of living in the fattest nation in the world, Americans continue to value thinness over more important character qualities, like honesty, integrity, and even intelligence.

Helping Your Overweight Child Lose Weight

If your overweight child is a toddler or preschooler, implementing healthy changes in your family's diet and exercise routine may not be all that difficult. Young children are very adaptive and likely to go with the flow, as long as their parents are supportive and willing to join in. Teenagers, on the other hand, are not quite as accommodating, and changes in the family routine may be met with a little more resistance.

There are a few steps mothers can take to make the transition to a healthier lifestyle a little smoother. First, moms should focus on improving

BMI for Adults

To determine your Body Mass Index, locate your height in the far left column of the chart. Look along the line of weight boxes to the right of your height and find the weight box closest to your weight. Next, look down at the very bottom of the column that your weight box is in. That's your BMI.

Height (inches)	Body Weight (pounds)																
58	91	96	100	105	110	115	119	124	129	134	138	143	148	153	158	162	167
59	94	99	104	109	114	119	124	128	133	138	143	148	153	158	163	168	173
60	97	102	107	112	118	123	128	133	138	143	148	153	158	163	168	174	179
61	100	106	111	116	122	127	132	137	143	148	153	158	164	169	174	180	185
62	104	109	115	120	126	131	136	142	147	153	158	164	169	175	180	186	191
63	107	113	118	124	130	135	141	146	152	158	163	169	175	180	186	191	197
64	110	116	122	128	134	140	145	151	157	163	169	174	180	186	192	197	204
65	114	120	126	132	138	144	150	156	162	168	174	180	186	192	198	204	210
66	118	124	130	136	142	148	155	161	167	173	179	186	192	198	204	210	216
67	121	127	134	140	146	153	159	166	172	178	185	191	198	204	211	217	223
68	125	131	138	144	151	158	164	171	177	184	190	197	203	210	216	223	230
69	128	135	142	149	155	162	169	176	182	189	196	203	209	216	223	230	236
70	132	139	146	153	160	167	174	181	188	195	202	209	216	222	229	236	243
71	136	143	150	157	165	172	179	186	193	200	208	215	222	229	236	243	250
72	140	147	154	162	169	177	184	191	199	206	213	221	228	235	242	250	258
73	144	151	159	166	174	182	189	197	204	212	219	227	235	242	250	257	265
74	148	155	163	171	179	186	194	202	210	218	225	233	241	249	256	264	272
75	152	160	168	176	184	192	200	208	216	224	232	240	248	256	264	272	279
76	156	164	172	180	189	197	205	213	221	230	238	246	254	263	271	279	287
BMI	19	20	21	22	23	24	25	26	27	28	29	30	31	32	33	34	35

the health of the entire family rather than single out an overweight child as the target of her attentions. It's not a good idea to say something like, "Ashley's pediatrician says she's overweight. I guess that means we'll have to cut out desserts." You really don't have to say anything at all. When it's time for dessert, serve up a tempting fruit salad or low-fat pudding instead of items that are higher in fat and calories. If kids question your selection, you can tell them that you're trying out some new recipes that taste good as well as being good for them.

It's best not to alarm your older kids by announcing that you're planning to totally revamp their lives. Saying something like, "Okay, kids. Things are going to change around here" will probably provoke apprehension, or even rebellion. The best way to bring about positive changes is to introduce them gradually and subtly, with as little fuss as possible.

If your teen happens to notice the changes you've implemented, you can explain that you're trying to improve the health of the entire family. If the time isn't right, you can always fall back on the "I'm only trying to be helpful" routine. When he goes rummaging through the cabinets for potato chips and comes up empty-handed, you can say something like, "I thought you'd rather have some fresh fruit for a change." You can even try to inflict a little education on him: "You know, I didn't realize how much fat those potato chips had until I read the nutrition label. Apples don't have any fat, and they're loaded with vitamins." If your teen seems interested, you can continue to dazzle him with your nutritional savvy. If, on the other hand, his eyes glaze over like two Krispy Kreme doughnuts, you'll know you've slipped into your maternal lecturing mode, and it's time to give it a rest.

One of the best ways to help overweight children slim down is to use the principle of substitution. Instead of simply taking foods away, substitute nutritious ones for those that aren't. If your ravenous kids go rooting around the kitchen like truffle pigs and find dried fruit in the cookie jar, bottled water in the fridge, and frozen yogurt instead of gourmet ice cream in the freezer, they'll improvise. If they're not all that hungry, they'll simply do without. Either way, you both win. As long as kids can find something tasty to munch on when they're hungry, they'll be more likely to give up the junk food without waging a major war. By keeping your kitchen stocked with a variety of nutritious foods, you can exert some measure of control over your children's eating behaviors without ever saying a word.

While you're helping your child build a healthy diet and establish a more active lifestyle, it's important to work on bolstering her self-esteem. It's important for moms to address children's concerns about weight, but it's not a good idea to use words like "fat" or "obese" when discussing them. Giving a child a negative label can be very damaging. If a child considers herself to be "fat" or "obese," she might end up adopting the destructive self-fulfilling prophecy that goes along with it.

You should also make sure that siblings don't tease your overweight child or call her derogatory names based on her weight. Reassure your child that you love and accept her just as she is, regardless of her weight. Focus on her positive character qualities and let her know that her weight does not determine her worth.

Unsafe Weight-Loss Practices

Children, especially adolescents, feel an enormous amount of pressure to be attractive. In our culture, being attractive means being thin. Studies show that 40 percent of American adolescents are currently trying to lose weight, and 30 percent are actively dieting. For teens, "dieting" can involve some drastic measures.

Since adolescents tend to diet in an effort to improve appearance rather than health, the use of unsafe weight-loss practices is extremely common. Overweight kids may turn to "quick fixes," such as self-induced vomiting or the use of diet pills, laxatives, and diuretics. Although obese and overweight girls are most likely to resort to these dangerous tactics, obese and overweight boys are known to try them as well. Teens who use these weight-loss strategies are at higher risk for engaging in other behaviors that compromise their health, including substance abuse, unsafe sexual behaviors, suicide attempts, and eating disorders.

Teens at greatest risk for using drastic and risky weight loss techniques are those with low self-esteem and those who don't understand how proper nutrition and regular exercise work in terms of promoting weight loss. This is where moms can step in and make a big difference. Teaching your children how to choose nutritious foods and engage in activities that promote weight loss allows them to make better decisions about fad diets and unsafe weight-loss practices.

Diets Don't Work

One of the worst things you can do to "help" your child lose weight is to put her on a diet. Coping with a weight problem is likely to be a lifelong challenge, and at best, dieting is a short-term solution. More often, it is the first step of what will become a self-defeating cycle. Temporary changes in eating habits can only bring about temporary weight loss. Even after successfully losing weight, the typical dieter can expect to regain all of the lost weight within one year—plus an additional fifteen pounds of bonus weight. To achieve permanent weight loss, kids must learn to make permanent changes in their lifestyles.

For kids, dieting is risky business. Their rapidly growing bodies depend on an adequate number of calories on a daily basis for proper development. Placing your child on a low-calorie or very low-fat diet may deprive her of the nutrients she needs at a critical time in her life, and it may even jeopardize her health.

Low-calorie diets are dangerous for another reason. Weight that is rapidly lost comes primarily from the body's muscle tissue rather than fat deposits. It's an unfortunate phenomenon, but it's inevitable. Muscle tissue is a metabolic inferno, and it churns up a lot of calories, even while the body is at rest. Body fat, on the other hand, is metabolically comatose. Even during strenuous exercise, body fat burns very few calories. If children lose even a pound or two of their precious muscle tissue on a low-calorie diet, they'll end up needing fewer calories each day than they did before the diet.

While weight-loss diets are physically harmful to growing children, they can also inflict some serious emotional damage. Strict diets are likely to create feelings of deprivation in children, and these feelings can eventually lead to overeating and binge eating.

Instead of putting your child on a low-calorie diet, your best bet is to show her how to eat properly. Teach her about the nutritional values of different foods and how to design a nutritious, well-balanced meal. If your child simply masters the art of eating the way she *should* be eating, dieting really isn't necessary. As your child becomes more active and continues to grow, she'll gradually lose her excess weight.

Physical Activity

While you're shaping up your kids' eating behaviors, remember that good nutrition is only half of the weight-loss equation. Exercising is equally important.

Keeping kids active takes a little extra effort on Mom's side. You may have to spend more time carting your children back and forth to soccer games, gymnastics, or karate classes. But they won't be kids forever, and the time to get them involved in fitness is while they're still young and willing to learn. If you don't help your kids develop the interest and the ability to engage in some type of exercise as youngsters, chances are slim that they'll pick it up in adulthood.

One of the best ways to get your kids to become more active is to become more active yourself. No matter how exhausted you are when you come home from work, you need to prod yourself into action, at least for a half hour or so. You can't really expect your kids to exercise if you're not willing to. The days of parental dictatorship are long gone. Our enlightened and empowered children are much more sophisticated than we were as kids, and they just aren't falling for the old "because I said so" routine.

Moms must model the behaviors they want to see in their children, and this applies to exercise as well as other areas of life. When you get up and get moving, your kids are likely to join you. If you show kids that exercise can be fun, you're giving them the lifelong gift of fitness.

Teach Kids To Be Self-Sufficient

Moms need to teach their children to fend for themselves in the kitchen. By encouraging them to help out at mealtime, you're giving them the skills they need to select and prepare nutritious foods when you're not there to do it for them.

Young kids love to be included in "grown-up" tasks, like pouring and measuring ingredients or washing and trimming fruits and vegetables. As you work together with your children, explain the nutrient value of each food and how it fits into a well-balanced diet. Also, if you teach your children how to use kitchen appliances and utensils safely, they'll be much less likely to burn the house down or injure themselves when you're not around to supervise.

You can keep mealtime interesting by allowing your kids to participate in meal planning. Encourage them to design menus, choosing a favorite food for each meal. Take your children with you to the supermarket to buy the ingredients you'll need. As you shop, you can discuss the choices you make. By reading nutrition labels on packages, you can compare the contents and nutritional value of different foods and different brands.

For teens who wouldn't be caught dead grocery shopping with their mothers, you may have to use a different approach. Try putting your older child in charge of meals once a week or so. Allow her to prepare her favorite dishes and experiment with new ones. If you teach your kids the skills they need to become self-sufficient in the kitchen, they'll be less likely to resort to diets consisting entirely of fast food and processed foods when they grow up.

Just as you and your children plan your meals, you should also plan your television consumption. Encourage kids to limit their TV time to an hour or two a day, and decide on a plan to make it work. Sit down with your kids and make a TV viewing schedule a week at a time, allowing each child to select a favorite show or two. As long as they're still able to catch their favorite shows, kids won't be as reluctant to give up some of their viewing time.

Real Moms Are Role Models

As a mother, you can help your children succeed at losing weight by making it very difficult to fail. You must give them the tools they need to succeed. While it's important to provide education, motivation, and support, you also have to pay attention to the details. Kids need ways and means to eat properly and exercise, including having access to a variety of nutritious foods and safe activities.

More than anything, kids need a mentor. You can't expect your children to change their eating and exercising habits if you're not willing to do the same. As a mother, you must lead kids with your own positive example. It takes some hard work and determination, but it's well worth the effort. By serving as a role model for your kids, you're helping them build the foundation they need for a lifetime of good health.

Chapter 3

Early Eating

Obesity in children is much easier to avoid than to treat, and prevention begins with the most important person in your child's life: you. Prevention of obesity actually starts in early infancy with the establishment of a positive feeding relationship between mother and child. This requires that you learn to recognize your infant's cues of hunger and satiety, provide foods that are developmentally appropriate and nutritionally sound, and make mealtime peaceful and enjoyable for yourself and your baby.

Preventing Obesity in Infancy

One of the best things you can do to start your baby off on the right nutritional path is to breastfeed. Breastfeeding has been shown to help prevent obesity in childhood and adolescence to a significant degree.

Dozens of studies have shown that newborns who are breastfed for the first six months of life are dramatically less likely to become obese than formula-fed babies. The risk appears to be even lower for babies who continue to nurse for seven months or more. The longer an infant is breastfed, the greater the protective effects against obesity, and the longer those effects last.

Children who are predominantly fed mothers' milk during the first six months of life have a lower prevalence of overweight and obesity throughout childhood, even nine to fourteen years later. Compared with infants that are fed commercial formula, the estimated reduction in risk is approximately 22 percent.

There are several schools of thought about why breastfed infants are less likely than formula-fed babies to become overweight later in life. One theory is that breastfed infants have more control over their food intake and thus their calorie consumption. They tend to nurse as long as they're hungry, and they promptly stop when their full bellies tell them that they've had enough. As a result, breastfed babies rarely overeat.

Formula-fed babies, on the other hand, have less control over their food intake, while their mothers have more. Many conscientious moms encourage their babies to finish the entire contents of the bottle at each feeding, especially after they went to the trouble of preparing it.

Also, infant formula is pretty pricey these days, and most moms find it economically prudent to feed it to their babies—whether they want it or not—rather than pour it down the drain. For this reason, moms may push their newborns to keep eating, even when their babies have indicated that they are full.

Nursing infants consume fewer calories at each feeding than those who are bottle-fed for still another reason. Breastfed babies consume 80 to 90 percent of the milk that they drink in the first four minutes of nursing, and this milk is relatively high in water content. The "hind milk" that follows is richer in fat and calories, but it is consumed in much smaller quantities, after the baby's hunger has been largely satisfied. Formula-fed babies, on the other hand, get a steady flow of milk that is uniform in fat and calorie content throughout the first ten minutes of feeding.

Another theory holds that the protective effect of breastfeeding against obesity could involve the metabolic consequences of consuming breast milk. Mothers' milk contains substances that seem to limit the number and size of fat cells in newborn babies.

Blood tests in infants reveal lower concentrations of insulin in breastfed babies than in formula-fed babies. Insulin is a hormone that promotes fat storage in the body, and the higher insulin levels of bottle-fed babies suggest that they have a greater capacity to store energy in the form of body fat.

There is little doubt that breastfeeding helps protect infants from becoming overweight or obese later in life, but the practice of nursing newborns is important for other reasons.

Not surprisingly, breast milk is the perfect food for babies. Its natural components are easily broken down and absorbed by infants' immature digestive systems. Mothers' milk is loaded with vitamins, minerals, and other nutrients required for the proper growth and development of newborns. It provides babies with enzymes and antibodies that they aren't able to produce themselves and protects them against the development of food and environmental allergies as they grow older.

With this in mind, the American Medical Association and the American Academy of Pediatrics recommend that babies be fed mothers' milk exclusively for the first four to six months of life and that breastfeeding be continued beyond the first birthday, if possible.

Mothers get a few bonus benefits for themselves if they choose to nurse their newborns. Mothers' milk is, for the most part, free. It is far less expensive than commercial baby formula, which can set new parents back about $1,500 in the first year of a baby's life.

Nursing your infant means that you always have a convenient, instantly accessible food supply. It relieves you of the unpleasant task of preparing and heating bottles in the middle of the night. Lactation also triggers muscular contraction of the uterus, speeding its return to a normal size. Additionally, mothers who breastfeed their babies burn a lot of calories in the process of producing milk, making it a little easier to shed extra postpartum pounds. Best of all, breastfeeding lowers a woman's risk of developing breast cancer later in life.

Breastfeeding for the working mom represents a unique challenge, as any woman who has tried it can tell you firsthand. This may be the reason that so many career women decide not to nurse their infants in the first place or choose to stop the practice prematurely. Most working moms return to work after just three months of maternity leave, and for many women, this seems to be a natural time to make the transition from nursing to formula feeding.

Mothers who continue to breastfeed while working are faced with the inconvenience—and sometimes the discomfort—of pumping their milk at work. It takes a very committed and determined mother to stick with the program in spite of it all.

I had the interesting experience of trying to juggle breastfeeding and the rigors of working after the birth of my third son. In order to maintain my status as a resident physician, "the powers that were" strongly encouraged me to return to work just a few short weeks after the blessed event.

Determined to continue breastfeeding in spite of the demands of my job, I humbly asked my supervising physician if he would allow me to take a short break every few hours to pump my milk. He agreed and hastily turned me over to his office manager to handle the details.

The office manager was a matronly, no-nonsense woman who had obviously borne her children at the height of the formula-feeding era. She immediately tried to dissuade me from my decision to nurse my child. It was quite apparent that she found the archaic practice of breastfeeding more suitable to hippies and tribal natives than to modern-day female physicians.

When it became obvious that I wouldn't be bullied into bottle-feeding, she marched me to a closet-sized bathroom at the back of the office building. Here, I would be hidden away from the more civilized members of society. The pint-sized lavatory would allow me to collect my milk in one of two positions: either standing in front of a mirror mounted above a tiny sink or sitting on the toilet, which unfortunately was not equipped with a lid.

I thanked the old prude anyway and asked her to kindly point me to a refrigerator where I could store my milk. She thought about my request for a minute and then led me to the medical office's laboratory, where she pointed to the industrial-sized, stainless steel refrigerator plastered with neon stickers proclaiming "Biohazard: Blood and Body Fluid!" This woman seriously expected me to store my hard-earned breast milk—the life-sustaining nectar of my precious baby boy—among stool samples, skin biopsies, and sputum cultures.

Looking back, I have to laugh, but my own experiences help me appreciate the fact that women who continue to breastfeed their infants after returning to work face some serious obstacles.

Working mothers who persevere in spite of the challenges will probably never regret the extra time and effort required of them. Most moms say that nursing their babies was one of the most rewarding and fulfilling experiences of their lives.

If your precious babies are now children or teenagers and you didn't breastfeed them in infancy, it's definitely too late to start now. But it is still helpful to understand why breastfeeding the newborn is so important. The principles that apply to breastfeeding also apply—at least in theory—to children of every age.

Demand Feeding

In infancy, moms should focus on learning to recognize their babies' signals of hunger and feed them accordingly. It's equally important to recognize signs of satiety. When baby's sucking becomes slow, when she turns her head away, or seems distracted or uninterested in the breast or bottle, it's time to stop feeding.

Whether you choose to nurse or bottle-feed, you should strive to avoid feeding your children too much, just as you strive to feed them enough. During infancy, mothers should master the art of demand feeding and become comfortable with it, as it will be useful throughout the remainder of the child's life.

There is little doubt that breastfeeding protects infants from becoming overweight and obese later in life, but whether newborns are fed from the breast or the bottle, overfeeding is still possible, and it can have harmful long-term effects. Studies in animals and humans indicate that overfed infants have greater numbers of fat cells, and those cells contain more fat than the cells of infants who are not overfed. These studies emphasize the importance of gauging and respecting your infant's appetite regardless of the means by which you choose to feed him.

Introducing Solid Foods

No matter how appealing it may seem, moms should strenuously resist the temptation to introduce solid foods to their babies until the fourth month of life, and preferably until the sixth month.

Mothers may feel a great deal of pressure to add solid foods to their babies' diets before they're truly ready for several reasons. One is the erroneous but common maternal notion that a heavy infant is a healthy infant. Many moms believe that having a chubby baby is a visible sign of successful feeding and thus successful parenting.

Another reason may be that many moms fear that their babies aren't getting enough to eat from the breast or the bottle. If mothers believe that their babies are inadequately nourished, they're more likely to turn to solid foods to fill in the caloric gaps.

Some moms push solid foods too early because they haven't learned that crying isn't always a sign of hunger. They think every infant cry is an indication of impending starvation, so they tend to poke bottles in their babies' mouths in response to every cry, grunt, or gurgle their cherished offspring emit. In many cases, however, babies' cries may represent something much more mundane, like boredom, loneliness, or a wet diaper.

Colicky babies tend to cry a lot, and not because they're hungry. Many mothers of colicky babies fear that their newborns are crying because they're hungry, and they introduce solid foods in an attempt to get a little more peace and quiet during the daytime, and a little more sleep at night. But as your pediatrician will assure you, introducing solid foods prematurely to colicky infants will only worsen the problem. In spite of popular myth, starting solid foods during the first few weeks of life really doesn't prolong the time between feedings, nor does it help babies sleep longer at night. Adding cereal to babies' formula isn't recommended either because babies can easily choke on the thickened liquid. Early consumption of solid foods adds unnecessary calories to babies' diets. Not only does this lead to rapid weight gain, but it also sets them up for a lifelong struggle with obesity. Another reason to hold off adding solid foods is that babies can develop allergies to foods when they're introduced too early in life. Their immature digestive systems just aren't capable of properly digesting solid foods before the age of four to six months.

When the time comes to introduce solid foods to their infants' diets, mothers who breastfed their babies will be glad they did. Breastfeeding seems to ease the transition from a liquid diet to one that contains solids.

As solid and finger foods are introduced to the growing infant, not all of them are accepted with great enthusiasm. This can be a time when struggles over feeding and eating begin. As a rule, breastfed infants tend to accept new and different foods more readily than formula-fed infants. The consumption of mothers' milk provides the infant with a smorgasbord of interesting flavors that varies with the mother's daily diet. Commercial formula, on the other hand, offers the baby a predictable, unvarying flavor across all feedings for the first several months of life. While breastfed babies are accustomed to accepting new and different tastes, formula-fed babies are not. This may present a challenge to mothers of bottle-fed infants, as they struggle to persuade their babies to eat a variety of nutritious foods that are necessary for a well-balanced diet.

Before you introduce solids to your baby, she should show several signs of readiness. First, she will have doubled her birth weight. She'll no longer seem satisfied after nursing or feeding from a bottle, and she'll become interested in the foods that everyone else in the family is eating. In order to eat solid foods safely, your baby should be able to sit up with a little support from you. She'll also be able to close her tiny lips around a baby spoon, and she won't grimace and reject the food with her tongue. She'll happily accept it, keep most of it in her mouth, and swallow it without gasping or choking.

Your baby's first spoonful of food is a very important and special event. In addition to strengthening the special bond between mother and child, it's an ideal time to introduce positive eating habits that will see your baby through a lifetime of good health. When the time is right to start your baby on solid foods, find a quiet time and place without distractions so that you can both concentrate on what you're doing. Using a baby spoon, offer your infant a small amount of food, wait for mouth to open—a sign that she's ready to move forward in the eating adventure—and gently spoon it in. Sit face to face with your baby and speak softly and reassuringly to her. Gently encourage her to taste new flavors and praise her for trying them. While moms should talk quietly to their babies during mealtime, it's not a good idea to try to entertain them or overwhelm them with attention or stimulation.

Offer your baby nutritious foods that are designed just for infants. Avoid giving her high-calorie foods and beverages like sodas, puddings, or desserts.

Allow her to touch—and even play with—her food if she wants to. It's a great way for her to explore the texture and consistency of what she'll be eating.

At each meal, babies should be allowed to eat at their own pace, and they should be allowed to stop when they indicate that they've had enough. Sure signs of dwindling appetites include turning away from food, fussiness, and sudden interest in something other than the task at hand.

If your infant seems famished before mealtime, offer him a small amount of breast milk or formula first to take the edge off his hunger. This will keep him from getting frustrated when solid food is too cumbersome to consume quickly and also reduce the chances that he'll choke on it.

When you're introducing solids to your baby's diet, iron-fortified rice cereal is one of the best foods to start with. It should be mixed with breast milk or formula to a thin, watery consistency. You can increase the thickness over time, after baby has become accustomed to eating solid foods. A week or so after rice cereal has been introduced and accepted, babies are usually ready for other single cereals, like oatmeal or barley. Once these foods have been conquered, it's time to move on to mixed cereals.

It's important to introduce only one new food every three to five days. At this pace, the baby's sensitive gastrointestinal system has time to adjust to the change in diet. It will also give you a chance to watch for any signs of adverse reactions to the new food, like diarrhea, vomiting, or a skin rash.

After cereals, pureed or strained vegetables like sweet potatoes, carrots, and peas should be offered, but only one at a time. Fruits should be introduced only after vegetables, since the sweet flavors of fruit can make the blander taste of vegetables seem far less appealing. Meat is generally best introduced at about seven to nine months of age.

If your baby refuses to eat a new food, just offer it again in a few days. Research indicates that it may take as many as ten to twelve failed attempts before an infant will finally accept a new flavor. Within a few weeks of introducing solids, most babies will eat several types of food at each meal for a total of roughly one-third to a half cup of cereal and up to a cup and a half of fruits and vegetables each day.

While you and your baby are working on building a nutritious diet, it's important to continue to offer milk on a regular basis. From four to six months of age, breast milk or formula is still necessary for your baby's proper growth and development, and solid food should never be used to replace either. Throughout infancy and the first year of life, all children should see their pediatricians regularly so that their health and weight can be monitored.

Preventing Obesity in Toddlers

As your child approaches the age of two years, it's up to you to set the stage for a lifetime of healthy eating habits. Start at the top, with you and the other members of your family serving as good examples. You really can't ask your toddler to eat properly if you do not. It's hard to imagine that your two-year-old will be excited about eating carrot sticks and celery while you sit by and munch on potato chips.

The American Academy of Pediatrics cautions against restricting children's intake of calories and fat before the age of twenty-four months. Toddlers are actively growing, and by limiting their consumption of calories and fat, you can end up negatively affecting their growth and development. Beginning at the age of two, it is acceptable for children to consume fewer calories from fat. Most healthy toddlers can safely limit their intake of fat to 30 percent of their total caloric intake. Moms can now replace whole milk and whole milk dairy products with 2 percent milk or skim milk and low-fat dairy products. The transition to a lower-fat diet should be gradual rather than sudden or strict, and if your toddler is underweight, you might want to hold off limiting fat intake for another year or so.

At the same time that toddlers make the transition to a lower-fat diet, they should begin to increase their consumption of nutrient-rich solid foods, like grains, fruits, and vegetables. Moms should make sure that toddlers are getting adequate amounts of fiber in their diets. As a general rule of thumb, kids should get 1 gram of fiber for each year of their age, plus 5 grams, up to a maximum of 25 to 30 grams of fiber each day. With this in mind, you would want to be sure a five-year-old child got at least 10 grams of fiber a day, while a seven-year-old would require at least 12 grams of fiber a day. Studies have shown that kids who eat high-fiber diets consume less fat and are less likely to be overweight than kids whose diets are low in fiber.

As toddlers struggle with issues of separation, autonomy, and limits, they can become amazingly obstinate. With their increasing independence and mobility, they become more physically active. As their appetites decrease and their need for independence grows, their food intake typically becomes erratic and unpredictable. This is the time when many moms become concerned about their children's lack of attention to eating and to food in general. They often blame their toddlers' declining rate of weight gain on their finicky appetites.

It is at this age that some moms unwittingly begin to instill negative food associations and bad eating patterns in their children. They often use food for non-nutritive purposes and employ strategies like bribery, punishment, or rewards to get their children to eat, or even to behave. It's not uncommon to hear an exasperated and desperate mother beseech an unruly tot to cooperate by saying things like "Sweetie-pie, if you'll just be still while Mommy finishes her shopping, we'll stop and get a milkshake on the way home."

You may have found yourself resorting to these very words from time to time. Moms must tread very lightly when it comes to rewarding toddlers with food. At the same time, moms should be cautious about withholding food as a punishment. It's just as damaging to say things like "If you don't sit still, you won't get any cookies for snack."

The use of food for non-nutritive purposes, like bribery, punishment, or reward, has both immediate and long-term negative consequences. It leaves children with a poor ability to recognize their own signals of hunger and satiety and makes it difficult for them to regulate their own food intake.

The inappropriate use of food removes the control of eating behaviors from the internal source (the child), where it should be, to a locus outside of the child (the child's mother), where it should not be. It ultimately leads to poor eating habits, putting the youngster at risk for childhood obesity, as well as a lifelong struggle with weight problems.

Because they're worried about their children's eating habits, many moms often make the mistake of preparing whatever foods their children request, whenever they want them. Fulfilling the desires of a demanding child is *not* the same as demand feeding. Nonetheless, many moms are overly accommodating to their children's whims. They rationalize their enabling behaviors with the thought that "at least they're not going hungry."

Concerns about a child's poor appetite or picky eating may also be the reason some mothers allow their children to continue taking a bottle long after the time for weaning has come and gone. It's bad enough to allow toddlers to continue bottle-feeding, but filling those bottles with high-calorie juices or sodas is even worse. Prolonged bottle-feeding not only contributes to childhood obesity, it also promotes tooth decay and the development of other dental problems.

Remember, "normal" growth for toddlers occurs at a much slower pace than it did during infancy. During the first twelve months of life, a weight gain of twelve to fifteen pounds is the norm. Between the ages of three to five years, however, a healthy child may not gain more than four pounds a year. That boils down to about a third of a pound per month, which may help you to relax a little when your child clams up and refuses to eat. A slower rate of growth helps explain why toddlers and preschoolers seem to have less than hearty appetites and display less interest in food.

By the time your child is a toddler, you must be prepared to relinquish a certain amount of control over his eating behaviors. Remember the golden rule of feeding your child: Mothers are responsible for serving a wide variety of nutritious foods to their children in a relaxed and comfortable environment. The decisions about how much to eat, and even whether to eat, belong entirely to the child.

Toddlers are beginning to join the rest of the family at mealtime, and this provides an excellent opportunity for moms to select and prepare a healthy diet for the entire family. In toddlers, the focus should be on instilling positive food associations, developing good eating habits, and building a varied and nutritious diet.

Moms should serve small amounts of soft, nutritious foods and provide at least two healthy snacks every day. Foods should be offered in shapes and sizes that your children can handle with their small mouths and fingers.

It's a good idea to introduce new foods regularly, but at every meal or snack, you should always include at least one familiar item that you know your child likes. By offering your child a new food, but not forcing her to eat it, you're allowing her to maintain her freedom of choice while expanding her dietary horizons.

If new food is offered, and the child decides she doesn't like it, at least there's something nutritious on the table that she *will* eat. This gives Mom the comfort of knowing that her child won't starve. It also prevents her from having to jump up from the table to prepare an additional dish that she knows her child likes. Giving in to requests or demands for "special" foods that aren't on the menu is a bad habit to develop—both for you and your child.

If your child refuses to eat the new foods *and* the old familiar standby at a given meal, that's fine. Moms should resist the temptation to bribe or beg their kids to eat, and they should never punish them for not eating. If little Jeffrey refuses to eat, he should be required to remain at the table until the rest of the family has finished dining. Only then may he be excused to attend to what he deems more pressing tasks.

After a less than successful meal, it's generally best to wipe the slate clean and start all over again. If your child comes to you in an hour claiming he's starving, it's okay to gently remind him that he wouldn't be starving if he had eaten his dinner. You don't have to go to a lot of trouble preparing his favorite food, but it's probably not a good idea to withhold food altogether. Eventually, your child will figure out that he's much better off enjoying the meal with the rest of the family.

You can comfort yourself with the knowledge that no matter how little food your child may consume at a given meal or even on a given day, starvation and malnutrition are virtually nonexistent among children who are routinely offered a balanced selection of nutritious foods. When you examine your child's diet, be sure to review his food intake over a period of several days, rather than just one meal or a single day. Kids may not eat everything you want them to every day of the week, but over the course of several days, they usually will manage to build a complete and well-balanced diet.

If you're still worried about your toddler's appetite and eating behaviors, be sure to discuss your concerns with your child's pediatrician. If the doctor feels that your child is growing and gaining weight in an acceptable pattern, you can rest assured that he's getting plenty to eat.

Preventing Obesity in Preschoolers

The preschool years are the time when kids show initiative, rebellion, and an eagerness to learn. At this age more than any other, a child's eating habits and food preferences are most influenced by his parents. Moms need to continue to model good food choices and eating behaviors.

In preschoolers, as in toddlers, fat should be limited to no more than 30 percent of the daily diet. Of the fat that preschoolers consume, no more than 10 percent should be fat of the saturated variety, according to the American Academy of Pediatrics.

Moms should pay attention to the quantities of food that their children are consuming. A general rule of thumb is to use approximately 1 table-spoon of food for each year of age for each portion served. This applies to fruits, vegetables, protein foods, and, when they are occasionally served, desserts. A snack for your three-year-old might consist of 3 tablespoons of applesauce, a few crackers, and a small glass of low-fat or skim milk.

When kids are outside of their home territory, it's not at all uncommon for them to scarf up foods that they usually reject. Studies show that when preschool children are given the opportunity to observe other kids choosing and eating vegetables that they themselves normally disliked and refused to eat, their intake of the previously disliked vegetable increases significantly.

What you serve your kids and what they actually eat may be two entirely different things. By offering your toddler a broad selection of nutri-tious foods from the five basic food groups, you're educating them about the importance of good nutrition and introducing them to a variety of deli-cious choices. You're also giving them the tools they'll need to construct good habits that will see them through a lifetime of good health.

Remember that as the mom, you are responsible for serving a variety of wholesome, nutritious foods in a pleasant atmosphere. It is up to your child to decide what and how much food to consume.

The Food Guide Pyramid for Young Children, developed by the U.S. Department of Agriculture, can help guide you in the appropriate food

Food Guide for Children Ages 2 to 6

Food Group	Number of Servings
Bread, cereal, rice, and pasta (mostly whole grain)	6 to 11
Vegetables	3 to 5
Fruits	2 to 4
Milk, yogurt, cheese, and low-fat dairy products	2 to 3
Meat, poultry, fish, dry beans, eggs, and nuts	2 to 3
Fats, oils, and sweets	Sparingly

choices and the recommended number of servings. The Pyramid is targeted to children aged two to six years. Your child's nutritional needs are best met by a balanced diet with a wide variety of foods from the basic food groups, served in age-appropriate portions. The proportions needed from each food group are the same as those for adults.

Picky Eaters

While there are no official medical criteria for the picky eater, you'll know if you have one. During the toddler and preschool years, picky eaters are the norm, rather than the exception. Foods can fall in and out of favor with amazing speed and for no apparent reason. Food jags are extremely common in this age group. Almost every child becomes devoted to a particular food at some point in time, steadfastly refusing to eat almost anything else.

In some cases, a certain degree of selectivity is protective for children. Some kids may instinctively avoid certain foods because they've learned that they don't feel well after eating them. If your child doggedly refuses to drink milk, it may be because he has a mild allergy to dairy foods or even lactose intolerance. You can still meet your child's need for dietary calcium by offering dairy foods that are more easily digested and better tolerated, like yogurt or cheese.

Coping with a picky eater can try the patience of any mother, but you can take comfort in the knowledge that finicky appetites rarely affect a child's health. With your continued effort and patience, plus a little tincture of time, even the pickiest kids will eventually assume a more normal pattern of eating.

Preventing Obesity in School-Aged Children

When children start elementary school, they enter an age of newfound independence and take a great deal of pride in being "big kids." They are enormously influenced by their friends and the media, and they have much more access to fast food and junk food.

As school-aged children mature into teens, they no longer eat all—or even most—of their meals at home. They seem to be hungry all the time, and because they're less inclined to eat clearly defined meals, they have a greater tendency to graze throughout the entire day. The easy availability of high-calorie foods and a growing tendency toward sedentary activities, like playing video games, talking on the telephone, and watching television, increase the risk of obesity in children of this age group.

Now, more than ever, moms must take the time and make the effort to stock the kitchen with an assortment of nutritious foods and snacks. Moms need to drastically limit the selection of high-calorie and high-fat foods in their homes, and make plenty of fruits, vegetables, and whole-grain foods available and appealing.

Mothers should continue to discourage TV dining, keeping the living room or television room off limits for eating. They must master stress-relieving techniques that don't involve eating and teach their children and teens to do the same.

Teens are often dismayed to find their bodies changing rapidly and dramatically, and they typically react to those changes in appearance with concern and confusion. Influenced by the media, most teenage girls become increasingly worried about their weight status. One study found that while 70 percent of teenage girls wanted to lose weight, only about 15 percent of them were too heavy. The same study found that while 59 percent of teenage boys longed to gain weight, only 25 percent of them were too thin.

Kids who are struggling with weight and body-image issues are at risk for developing eating disorders and engaging in dangerous weight-loss techniques, like fasting or using laxatives or diet pills. Moms need to focus on maintaining their kids' positive self-image and bolstering their self-esteem. Normal-weight teens need to be reassured that the changes in their bodies, as well as the feelings they're experiencing about them, are perfectly normal. Overweight teenagers who want to lose weight should be encouraged to focus on proper eating habits and regular exercise rather than on questionable weight-loss strategies.

Mothers should continue to try to coordinate the busy schedules of every member of the family, rounding teens up for regular family meals as often as possible. In spite of the inevitable parent-teen conflicts, the dinner table should never be allowed to serve as a battlefield. By ensuring that mealtime is a sacred period of familial truce, you will keep it a pleasant, positive experience. Any disagreements, arguments, or criticisms should be put aside whenever the family gathers around the table to break bread.

During the teen years, kids gain the final 20 percent of their adult height and the final 50 percent of their adult weight. Despite their increasing nutritional needs, these children are the least likely of all age groups to eat a well-balanced diet. The wide rebellious streak that typifies the average teen makes it very difficult for mothers to impose any type of dietary guidance.

The good news is that if you've instilled sound eating practices in your offspring before the teen years strike, he'll be more likely continue to eat well as a teenager. Lapses in dietary discretion are likely to be infrequent and short-lived, and your teenage nutritional delinquent will undoubtedly return to his former style of eating as he matures.

Chapter 4

The Four Critical Hours

Nutritionally speaking, afternoons represent a four-hour danger zone for children, especially when they're home alone, without the benefit of maternal supervision. Most kids consume up to a third of their daily calories in the hours between school dismissal and suppertime. Compounding the problem of a four-hour grazing spree, the after-school hours are often the time of greatest inactivity for kids, who typically spend much of them vegged out in front of television sets or plugged into computers or PlayStations.

Not only are latchkey kids more likely to have weight problems than kids who come home to a parent or sitter, they also face other dangers to their health. Studies have shown that kids with too much unsupervised time on their hands demonstrate more delinquent behaviors, like smoking and drinking alcohol. Long, solitary hours watching TV means less time spent interacting and building relationships with other people and can lead to social isolation and loneliness.

The Couch Potato Epidemic

The escalation of childhood obesity has some common culprits that keep kids in a near-comatose state on the couch and off the playground. The greatest offender is television, and not far behind are TV's technological cousins, computers and video games.

In the past fifty years, kids' access to the media has exploded, beginning with the introduction of television, which is now a permanent fixture in 98 percent of American households. In the early eighties, cable blasted into American homes, bringing with it MTV and twenty-four-hour cartoon networks. Additional youth-oriented channels kept kids glued to the tube, with little time left for playing or exercising. In the same era, tender young sofa spuds across the nation rejoiced as videocassette recorders and remote control devices made their debut. Changing channels became as effortless as lifting a single finger, making it easier than ever to remain couched for hours at a stretch. As the selection of channels continues to expand, and as parents grow increasingly dependent on the electronic box to serve as a bargain babysitter for their children, the negative consequences of owning a television set worsen.

For the past fifteen years, the American Academy of Pediatrics and other organizations have voiced their concerns about the amount of time kids spend watching television. Television viewing has become the number-one leisure-time "activity" among kids, and they spend a substantial part of their lives engaged in this favorite hobby. On a daily basis, the average American child spends about four to five hours watching television, for a grand total of twenty to thirty hours a week. Over a third of kids watch more than five hours a day. A recent study based on Nielsen Media Research data revealed that between the ages of two and seventeen, U.S. children spend an average of more than three years of their waking lives watching television. The typical high school graduate will probably have spent 15,000 to 18,000 hours in front of a TV set, but only 12,000 hours in school. By the time this child reaches the age of seventy, he will have spent the equivalent of seven to ten years of his life watching TV—enough time to complete college and earn a master's degree.

These figures don't include time spent watching videotapes, playing video or computer games, or surfing the Net. The emergence of personal computers, videocassette players, and video games has dramatically increased the amount of time kids spend suspended in a state of virtual inertia. A recent study found that U.S. kids while away an average of six hours and thirty-two minutes per day with various types of media combined. As the second most popular form of childhood recreation after television, video games have rapidly become the largest segment of the entertainment industry. They currently account for approximately 30 percent of toy market sales in the U.S., with nearly 200 million computer games sold each year. About 90 percent of American households with kids own or regularly rent video computer games.

Boys tend to spend more time playing video games than girls. Sixty percent of American girls log an average of two hours weekly on video players, while 90 percent of boys play for more than four hours per week. When kids sit down in front of video stations, it's usually for more than just a quick game: they typically play for one to three hours at a time. Although playing time generally slacks off as grade level increases, this sedentary pursuit follows most kids into young adulthood. Ninety-seven percent of college students admit to playing video games on a regular basis.

Tube Time and Obesity

While most kids have easy access to televisions, computers, and video games, some youngsters have virtually *unlimited* access. An estimated 40 percent of American children have televisions in their bedrooms, and nearly half have video game systems to go along with them. Both of these luxuries are strongly linked to childhood overweight and obesity; kids with a boudoir TV rack up an additional five hours of tube time each week. As a result, they are significantly more likely to be overweight than less "privileged" kids who are forced to hang out with their folks in the family room to watch television or play video games.

Studies show that the rate of obesity is highest in children and adolescents who watch more than four hours of television a day, while it is lowest in kids who watch less than an hour a day. Before the explosion of media options, most kids devoted their free time to more physical pursuits, like playing ball with other neighborhood kids, riding bikes, or doing strenuous chores. As the hours that modern-day kids spend watching television climb, time spent exercising declines dramatically, especially among girls.

A significant decrease in physical activity occurs as girls move from the eleven-to-thirteen-year-old age group to the fourteen-to-sixteen-year-old age group.

An Anti-Activity

Watching television isn't exactly labor-intensive. The number of calories expended during television viewing is practically zilch. In a recent study involving eight-to-twelve-year-olds, researchers found that, incredibly, kids' metabolic rates were significantly lower while watching TV than they were during periods of rest. Even fidgeting burns far more calories than sitting in a motionless, mesmerized state in front of the tube.

It shouldn't come as a big surprise that there is widespread speculation that television viewing, as part of a sedentary lifestyle, is one of the most easily modifiable causes of obesity among children. A recent Harvard study found that kids who rack up more than five hours of television viewing a day are nearly five times more likely to be overweight as those who watch two hours or less each day. Several other studies have demonstrated beyond a shadow of a doubt that the more time kids spend in front of television sets and computers, the more likely they are to be overweight and obese.

The American Academy of Pediatrics recommends that children's TV viewing time be limited to two hours or less each day and that programs be carefully reviewed and selected by parents for the appropriateness of their content. Sadly, studies find that only about 11 percent of American children meet this recommendation.

Surfing and Snacking

Watching too much television contributes to weight gain, but the problem is compounded when channel surfing is combined with snacking, a common practice among U.S. kids and adults. Folks tend to eat too much when they're sitting in front of the TV set, primarily because they pay more attention to what's on the tube than to what's in their stomachs. While they're tuned in to television, they're tuning out their internal signals of hunger and satiety, and they may not notice when their stomachs are telling them that they've had enough to eat. Several studies have shown that kids consume far more calories when they eat by themselves in front of the TV than they do when they sit down at the table and eat regular meals with their families.

The Commercial Trap

No matter how bad kids' television programs are, the commercials are likely to be worse. The barrage of food ads begins when babies are still in diapers, even when they're tuned in to public television channels. Shows like *Sesame Street* and *Teletubbies* are often underwritten by fast food franchises, so while kids are getting a little education via the airwaves, they're being force-fed a steady stream of mind-melting messages that undermine good eating habits and promote poor nutrition and weight gain.

Toddlers and young children aren't able to differentiate fully between what they see and hear on television and what they actually feel. When slick hucksters disguised as clowns, captains, and cute little animals tell them they're hungry for a specific type of junk food and the time to eat it is now, kids are likely to act on the suggestion. Until they reach the age of eight or nine, most children aren't even able to distinguish between the programs and advertisements. Lacking the bulletproof body armor of adult cynicism, young children believe almost everything they see and hear. When Michael Jordan says he eats at McDonald's every chance he gets, it never occurs to young kids that he might be exaggerating for the sake of financial gain. If they yearn to be like Mike, they'll naturally want to eat at McDonald's as often as possible.

Using shameless and seductive marketing ploys, manufacturers of kid-targeted junk foods have a huge negative impact on kids' food preferences and eating behaviors. They build the trap of obesity with sugary, fat-laden, high-calorie foods, and then lure kids into it using celebrity endorsements, toys, games, and contests as bait. Food advertisements account for roughly half of the commercials viewed by kids, and junk foods are among the most heavily advertised items on children's television programs. Nine out of ten foods advertised are high in fat, sugar, and calories. Only 2 percent of all advertisements paid for by food manufacturers sing the praises of fruits, vegetables, grains, or beans, and it shows on our nation's children. Most American children get about half of their daily caloric intake from fat and sugar that is added to foods, while only about 1 percent of all U.S. children eat diets that even remotely resemble the Food Guide Pyramid.

Businesses spend an estimated $13 billion a year marketing food and drinks to U.S. kids and their parents, a figure that has increased by nearly $5 billion in the past decade alone. By the time a food commercial makes its way into a child's mind via the television, market analysts and high-priced ad agencies have little doubt that their precisely aimed pitches will hit the mark. It's easy to understand why food manufacturers bypass parents and draw a bull's eye directly on children themselves. Spending by kids under the age of twelve tripled in the 1990s, reaching a staggering $23.4 billion in 1997. This figure doesn't include the billions of dollars' worth of junk food, fast food, and soft drinks that kids pestered their parents into buying for them.

With American kids smack-dab in the midst of an obesity epidemic, and with obesity now the second leading cause of death in the United States, you might think that Uncle Sam would wade into the food-advertising fiasco and take some action. The precedence has already been set with the ban of television ads for cigarettes and the restrictions that apply to televised beer commercials. But so far, it's a no go. Thankfully, Joe Cool and the Marlboro man are out, and Spuds McKenzie is on a very short leash, but Ronald McDonald is still hanging tough. The Federal Trade Commission made a valiant effort to regulate advertisements to kids in the 1970s, but they encountered a congressional roadblock that proved to be insurmountable. Since then, the number of kid-targeted food commercials has skyrocketed, and the rise in the number of overweight and obese children is following the same trend.

By the time the average American child reaches the age of eighteen, he will have viewed well over a million television commercials, and a large percentage of those will have featured high-pressure, brain-scrubbing messages to eat junk food and eat *lots* of it. For this reason alone, there's little wonder that the more television kids watch, the more fat and calories their diets contain, and the more overweight they are likely to be.

Setting TV Limits

It's tough for moms to compete with the continuous bombardment of slick advertising tricks and celebrity endorsements, but you don't have to rip the television cord from its socket to promote good health in your children. The simple act of turning off the television has been proven to help kids eat less, become more active, and lose weight, even if you do or say nothing else at all. Research has found that when the TV is off, kids naturally eat less and gravitate toward more physically demanding activities.

In a study in which kids were asked to do nothing more than to limit their television viewing to seven hours a week, weight loss was the result. Even without intentionally changing their eating or exercising habits, kids demonstrated significant decreases in Body Mass Index, waist circumference, and waist-to-height ratio.

If you're trying to limit kids' viewing time and be a little more selective about the programs they watch, you might want to try budgeting their TV time. You can start by giving your kids a television "allowance" of seven to twelve hours each week. At the beginning of each week, take a few minutes to sit down with your children and help them choose the shows that they most want to watch—and of which you're most likely to approve.

It's also a good idea to watch TV with your child from time to time and comment on the real messages delivered by programs and commercials. Help your kids understand the less than benevolent motivation behind the advertising schemes. Explain to them that the manufacturers of junk foods are much more concerned about corporate wealth than they are about kids' health.

Structured Afternoons

One way to keep kids off the computer and away from the television while you're not at home with them is to enroll them in after-school activities. School sports programs not only keep kids occupied during the critical afternoon hours, they also promote fitness and make weight control easier. Even if your child isn't interested in participating in team sports, he might be willing to join the school band, the student council, or the debate team.

If after-school programs aren't available or practical, you may need to reexamine your options. Some working moms are successful in persuading nearby relatives to get involved in their children's after-school care. You might find a reliable college student or a trustworthy retiree to oversee kids' afternoon activities and provide transportation when necessary. Your children may be able to ride the bus to a local YMCA, Boys & Girls Club, or gym after school a few days a week. Not only would these excursions provide them with a little adult supervision and physical activity, they would also limit their television and computer time.

If all else fails, you might even consider cutting your work schedule to part time so that you'll be home with your kids in the afternoons. Making arrangements to ensure that your children are supervised after school may be inconvenient at best, not to mention expensive. But if the extra effort and expenses help your kids stay active and healthy, you'll probably agree that the benefits far outweigh the costs.

If none of these options are possible or practical, there are a few steps you can take to keep your latchkey kids healthy and fit by helping them plan their afternoons. Without structure, bored and lonely kids are more likely to turn to TVs, computers, or video games in search of a little company and ready-made entertainment. Sit down with your child and write out a plan for the afternoon hours. You can use a dry-erase board, chalkboard, or poster to list activities that she can do while you're away from home. You might suggest that she kick back and relax for an hour or so after a long, hard day at school, then finish her homework, set the table, and make a salad. If she'll exercise on her own, you can schedule time for fitness. Offer to reward her for using her time alone productively by agreeing to take her on a window-shopping/fitness walk through the mall after dinner or joining her for a bike ride around the neighborhood.

Kids are more likely to exercise on their own when their homes are fitness-friendly. As the rumpus rooms of the past are being replaced with TV rooms and game rooms, modern-day kids have limited opportunities to engage in carefree indoor play. You don't have to spend a fortune on treadmills and exercise bikes to help your children stay fit at home. Kids are experts at making do with what they have to manufacture their own fun. Just provide them with a few essentials, such as balls, sidewalk chalk, skates, and jump ropes, and let the games begin!

It's important for kids to have designated places to romp and play, both inside and out. Move the cars out of the garage so that kids can jump rope, dribble basketballs, or jog on a mini trampoline. Rearrange the living room furniture so that kids can crank up their favorite music and practice their dance moves. Give your kids the go-ahead to set up a training course in the house, using stairs, chairs, and open floor space as fitness stations.

Action Plan

✔ **Remove bedroom TV sets.** If your child has a television set or computer in his bedroom, move it to a different location. Assure him that you're not punishing him; you're simply trying to foster family togetherness and fitness.

✔ **Make a TV viewing schedule.** Buy a *TV Guide* or similar directory, and sit down with your kids to plan the upcoming week's viewing schedule. Allow kids to spend their TV allowance on shows that meet your approval and write down their choices so that you can keep track of their TV time. If their favorite programs come on at inconvenient times, you can always tape them for later viewing.

✔ **Plan family fitness outings.** While you're all together in a planning mode, schedule a couple of family fitness outings for the week, like a picnic lunch, a nature walk, a bike ride, or a trip to the community swimming pool.

✔ **Promote educational programs.** Encourage your kids to watch programs that educate or build interest in other activities, like gardening or fitness.

✔ **Take interest in their favorite shows.** To show your kids that you care about their viewing habits, watch their favorite shows with them from time to time. Ask them what they like most about the characters and what they learn from the programs. If the program's values conflict with yours, discuss the reasons why with your kids.

✔ **Create an after-school plan.** With less time spent in front of the TV, your kids will have a lot more free time on their hands. Help them create a schedule for the hours after school and check to see how closely they follow it when you get home from work.

✔ **Establish priorities.** Don't allow kids to watch TV until they've completed their homework and finished their chores.

✔ **Make an after-school job box.** Write one simple task or activity on a slip of paper and attach a reward for its completion. For example, vacuuming the living room might be worth fifty cents, while the payoff for cleaning the bathroom might be a coupon good for one round of miniature golf.

✔ **Take your kids to the library.** Let them pick out a few fitness tapes and books to work out with when they're home alone.

✔ **Let them be the stars.** Show your kids how to operate the video recorder and allow them to make their own exercise tapes.

✔ **Praise their progress.** Be sure to praise your children for every step they take in the right direction, no matter how small or insignificant it may seem. Change happens slowly, and if kids think you don't notice their efforts, they're likely to stop trying.

Chapter 5

The G-Factor Program

If your pediatrician has officially pronounced your child overweight, you may react with surprise, dismay, or concern, but you'll definitely want to take positive steps to correct the problem. You don't have to take drastic measures, like having the poor child's jaws wired shut or forcing him to subsist on starvation rations until he slims down. The first thing to do is to remain calm. Remember that as your child matures, he will undoubtedly grow. If he's only moderately overweight, his height will eventually catch up to his weight, provided you help him avoid gaining more.

You, on the other hand, are an entirely different story. At this point in your life, you have probably already attained your maximum growth, at least in the vertical direction. If you're overweight, maintaining that weight is infinitely better than piling on additional pounds, but you'll undoubtedly benefit from a little weight loss.

The good news is that both you and your child can lose all the weight you need to without ever going on a diet. In fact, one of the worst things you can do to "help" your child lose weight is to put him on a diet. Most pediatricians strenuously recommend *not* putting children younger than eight on low-calorie or low-fat diets.

The Dangers of Restrictive Dieting

Restricting kids' intake of certain nutrients or the appropriate amount of food is always risky business. Children's rapidly growing bodies depend on an adequate number of calories on a daily basis for proper growth and development. Placing your child on a low-calorie or very low-fat diet may deprive him of the nutrients he needs at a critical time in his life, and it may even jeopardize his health.

Low-calorie diets are dangerous for another reason. Weight that is rapidly lost comes primarily from the body's muscle tissue rather than fat deposits. It's an unfortunate phenomenon, but it's inevitable. Muscle tissue is a veritable metabolic inferno, incinerating calories like a blast furnace, even while the body it inhabits is at rest. Body fat, on the other hand, is metabolically comatose. Even during strenuous exercise, body fat just sits there like a slug, burning hardly any calories at all. If you or your children end up sacrificing even a pound or two of precious muscle mass on a low-calorie diet, you'll end up needing far fewer calories each day than you did before you went on the diet. Loss of body muscle is responsible for the phenomenon of "rebound" weight gain that almost always occurs after rapid-weight-loss diets. Most dieters regain all of the lost weight plus an additional five to fifteen bonus pounds within a year of going on a diet.

Low-calorie diets also result in a slowing of the body's metabolic rate. This phenomenon is the result of a preprogrammed survival mechanism that remains in excellent working order even though it is now outdated and even unnecessary.

Back in the old days, and I'm talking about millennia ago, human beings ate heartily in times of plenty, and they nearly starved when times were lean. Over the centuries, the human body has become very adept at taking advantage of the plentiful times to ensure survival when food becomes scarce. When food was readily available and eaten liberally, the human body stored the excess energy in the form of body fat. In the event of a hard winter or a poor hunting season, body fat could be pulled out of storage and used as an alternative source of fuel.

If you fast-forward to modern-day America, you'll find that we no longer depend on these fat stores for survival. We can stock away enough food to live through a major famine in our industrial-sized, frost-free Frigidaires. But the human body hasn't caught on to this fact yet. It doesn't know how long the good times are going to last, so it continues to save more and more energy in the form of body fat, just in case. And its ability to store fat is virtually limitless. If it runs out of room, it just starts building additions, like spare tires, saddlebags, and double or triple chins.

If you're tired of adding on and want to slim down instead, you may decide to go on a diet and drastically reduce your caloric intake. While this seems perfectly logical, it's actually a big mistake. In response to what your body perceives as starvation, it switches into a survival mode and slams on the brakes of your metabolic machinery.

The metabolic rate is the rate at which your body burns calories. If you dramatically lower the number of calories you consume in the form of food, your body, fighting for your survival, reacts by burning fewer calories than before.

Low-calorie diets deliver a double whammy to your metabolism. In addition to promoting the loss of calorie-incinerating muscle mass, they also lower the metabolic rate itself. After this type of diet, your body needs significantly fewer calories to support itself than it did before. Studies have shown that some obese dieters have lowered their metabolic rates to the point where eating more than 1,000 calories a day actually results in weight gain.

In addition to being physiologically damaging, dieting is also emotionally damaging. By nature, humans always want what they can't have. Low-calorie diets instill feelings of suffering and deprivation, especially in children, who may not fully understand the reasons behind them. If you forbid your child to have a cookie, he may suddenly find himself wanting that cookie more than his next breath of air. Deprivation is the instigator of eating disorders, such as binge eating, as well as dangerous weight-loss practices, such as the use of laxatives or self-induced vomiting. While you and your child are losing weight, make sure that neither of you suffers from feelings of deprivation.

Coping with a weight problem is likely to be a lifelong challenge, and, at best, dieting is a short-term solution. More often, it is the first step of what will become a heartbreaking, self-defeating cycle. Temporary changes in eating habits can only bring about temporary weight loss. To achieve permanent weight loss, kids—and their parents—must learn to make permanent changes in their eating habits, and their lifestyles.

Diet Done Right

Although trying to follow or inflict the rigid rules and regulations of a diet is clearly the wrong way for you and your kids to lose weight, you still need some general guidelines about what and how much to eat for sound nutrition and good health. The best plan is one that doesn't require you to eat certain foods at certain times. If your family is trying to follow a diet that requires you to have a grapefruit half and a slice of whole-wheat toast for breakfast, you're going to run into some big problems sooner or later. What happens on the morning that you find that your last piece of whole-wheat bread has been invaded by a colony of mold? Or if your kids would rather eat stewed worms than choke down a slice of grapefruit? Situations like these usually cause dieters to can the diet and go right back to their old ways of eating.

The G-Factor Program (the G stands for "Grams") provides a sensible, flexible framework for you and your kids to get all the nutrients that your bodies need, in the proper proportions. While you're following the program, you can eat just about any food you like, as long as it falls within the guidelines. If your whole-wheat bread is toast, and your kids refuse to eat grapefruit, that's no problem. How about a nice, fresh slice of cantaloupe and a bagel instead? For busy moms and their kids, flexibility is a key ingredient for implementing lifestyle changes that last a lifetime, rather than just a few short weeks or months.

You and your children will be less likely to suffer feelings of deprivation when you're getting plenty to eat and satisfying your hunger. On the G-Factor Program, no foods are totally off limits. If you find yourself experiencing a nostalgic twinge of longing for a chocolate-covered, crème-filled doughnut, then it's okay to have one every now and then—as long as you don't eat the entire box. Periodically giving in to your cravings will make it easier to choose more nutritious foods on a regular basis.

To keep cravings to a minimum, it's important to stay focused on the positive aspects of your new way of eating, rather than the negative. Instead of grieving the loss of all the foods that you *can't* or *shouldn't* eat, think about all the delicious, nutritious foods that you will be eating. Remind yourself and your children of all the benefits that you'll enjoy, like higher energy levels, increased endurance and stamina, and a greater sense of self-esteem and self-confidence.

You'll encounter less resistance and get better results from your kids if you simply take the appropriate actions without making a big deal about it. Replacing foods that are high in fat and sugar with more nutritious ones that are loaded with vitamins, minerals, and fiber is an excellent place to start. The last thing you want to do is become a food cop. If you make the mistake of watching your kids like a hawk every time they eat, monitoring every morsel of food they nervously or defiantly place into their mouths, you'll practically doom them to failure. The best thing to do is to relax a bit and allow your kids to make their own choices about what to eat, within certain limits. The catch is that they'll only be able to choose from the foods that are available to them. In your own home, at least, you can make sure that the selection includes foods that support your new lifestyle.

Food Guide Pyramid

The G-Factor Program helps you and your kids get all the nutrients your bodies need while you lose weight. It complements the U.S. Department of Agriculture's Food Guide Pyramid, which is generally accepted by doctors and nutritionists as the gold standard of dietary recommendations. When you follow the Pyramid guidelines, you can be sure that you and your children are getting a nutritious, well-balanced diet.

The Food Guide Pyramid depicts the five major food groups, each of which provides some, but not all, of the nutrients you need each day. Foods at the base of the Pyramid are rich in complex carbohydrates and should be eaten in the greatest amounts, while those at the top of the Pyramid are high in fat and simple sugars and should be eaten in much smaller quanti-

Servings Needed Each Day

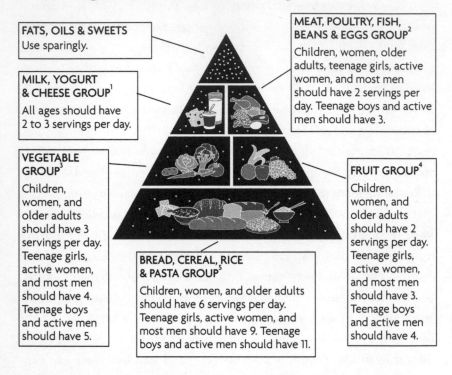

FATS, OILS & SWEETS
Use sparingly.

MILK, YOGURT & CHEESE GROUP[1]
All ages should have 2 to 3 servings per day.

MEAT, POULTRY, FISH, BEANS & EGGS GROUP[2]
Children, women, older adults, teenage girls, active women, and most men should have 2 servings per day. Teenage boys and active men should have 3.

VEGETABLE GROUP[3]
Children, women, and older adults should have 3 servings per day. Teenage girls, active women, and most men should have 4. Teenage boys and active men should have 5.

FRUIT GROUP[4]
Children, women, and older adults should have 2 servings per day. Teenage girls, active women, and most men should have 3. Teenage boys and active men should have 4.

BREAD, CEREAL, RICE & PASTA GROUP[5]
Children, women, and older adults should have 6 servings per day. Teenage girls, active women, and most men should have 9. Teenage boys and active men should have 11.

[1] **One serving from Milk, Yogurt & Cheese group** equals 1 cup (8 ounces) low-fat milk or yogurt; or 2 slices cheese (1½ ounces); or 2 cups cottage cheese; or 1½ cups ice milk, ice cream, or frozen yogurt.

[2] **One serving from the Meat, Poultry, Fish, Beans & Eggs Group** equals 2 to 3 ounces cooked lean meat, poultry, or fish (the size of a deck of cards); or 2 eggs; or 1 cup cooked legumes (dried beans or peas); or 4 tablespoons peanut butter; or ½ cup nuts or seeds.

[3] **One serving from the Vegetable Group** equals ½ cup raw chopped vegetables; or 1 cup raw leafy vegetables; or ½ cup cooked vegetables; or ¾ cup 100% vegetable juice.

[4] **One serving from the Fruit Group** equals 1 whole medium-sized piece of fruit; or ½ cup canned fruit; or ¼ cup dried fruit; or ½ cup 100% fruit juice.

[5] **One serving from the Bread, Cereal, Rice & Pasta Group** equals 1 slice bread; or 1 medium low-fat muffin; or ½ hot dog bun or hamburger bun; or ½ bagel or English muffin; or 1 cup cold cereal; or 4 small crackers; or 1 tortilla; or ½ cup cooked rice or pasta.

KEY: ◻ = Fats (naturally occuring and added)　▼= Sugars (added)

ties. If you're trying to lose weight, it's important to eat at least the minimum number of servings suggested in each of the five groups, rather than leave out an entire group altogether.

The Food Guide Pyramid gives a range of servings for each of the five major food groups. The number of servings that you need from each food group depends on the number of calories your body requires to maintain a desirable weight.

If the Food Guide Pyramid has one shortcoming, it's that it doesn't take into account the *actual amounts* of carbohydrates, proteins, and fats that a single serving of a particular food contains. Even when you're trying your best to follow the recommendations set forth by the Pyramid, you can still go astray. If, for example, you eat the two to four recommended servings from the "dairy" group, you might end up consuming too much fat. When you're trying to pack six servings from the breads group into your daily diet, you can easily exceed your allotment for simple carbohydrates. By applying the principles of the G-Factor Program to the Food Guide Pyramid, you'll be absolutely certain that you're getting a nutritious, well-balanced diet. The precise balance of carbohydrates, proteins, and fats in your diet will maximize your metabolic rate, enhance your energy levels, and make weight loss easier than you ever thought possible.

Keeping Track

While you're getting adjusted to your new way of eating, you might want to keep track of your daily intake by documenting each meal or snack. There's something about putting things on paper that keeps you honest, so this will help ensure that what you actually ate on any given day is roughly the same as what you intended to eat. Once you've mastered the G-Factor Program, choosing foods that support your new way of eating will be practically effortless. At this point, you can throw your pen and paper away and simply rely on your natural instincts to keep you on track.

The Three Key Nutrients

A balanced diet for kids and adults contains each of the three nutrients: carbohydrates, proteins, and fats. Although each nutrient is vital to your good health, their *combination* in your diet is of primary importance. The G-Factor Program allows you to balance carbohydrates, proteins, and fats in your daily diet in a very precise manner, with very little effort. This precise balance of nutrients not only makes for a well-rounded diet but also helps keep your hunger under control, boosts your metabolism, and dramatically enhances your weight loss.

1. Carbohydrates

Contrary to everything that you may have heard or read in the past few years, carbohydrates are *not* the dietary villains they've been made out to be. In fact, they're a very important part of your healthy diet—especially in terms of volume. They're so important that half of your daily caloric intake should come from carbohydrate-rich foods. If your daily diet consists of 2,000 calories, for example, 1,000 of those calories should come from carbohydrates.

Getting an adequate number of carbohydrates in your diet is important, but it's even more important to choose the right kinds. As it turns out, there are two types: *simple* carbohydrates and *complex* carbohydrates.

Sources of Carbohydrates

Good sources of complex carbohydrates include pasta, bread, rice, whole grain foods, cereals, and legumes. Simple carbohydrates, on the other hand, are abundant in foods like cookies, candies, and other sugary snacks. Believe it or not, many fruits and some types of vegetables, including carrots and potatoes, also fall into the simple carbohydrate category. Since you'll only be getting 20 percent of your carbohydrate calories from simple carbohydrate foods, it's important to make them count. Instead of wasting these calories on junk foods, you'll want to invest them in fruits and vegetables. Though they may contain simple carbohydrates, fruits and veggies are excellent sources of vitamins, minerals, and fiber, and you should strive to eat the recommended four to five servings every day.

Simple Carbohydrates

Both simple and complex carbohydrates are made up of smaller building blocks, and those building blocks are individual sugar molecules. In simple

Complex and Simple Carbohydrate Foods

Complex Carbohydrates

Whole grains: whole-grain breads and pasta, brown rice, oatmeal, cracked wheat, whole wheat, rye, barley

Legumes: lentils, garbanzo beans (chickpeas), navy beans, kidney beans, pinto beans, dried beans, peas

Cereals: bran, wheat, oatmeal

Simple Carbohydrates

Refined foods: white breads, cereals, pasta, cookies, cakes, pastries, candies

Soft drinks: sodas, sports drinks, punch, sugar-sweetened drinks

Fruit juices: 100% fruit juices, fruit "-ades" and "cocktails"

Sugars: table sugar, brown sugar, syrups, honey

---

carbohydrates, these sugar molecules are linked in a simple, linear fashion, with only a single bond between them. Because the bonds that hold simple carbohydrates together are very easily broken down in the digestive tract, they are quickly and easily converted back to sugar and almost instantly released into the bloodstream. When you eat a food made up of simple carbohydrates, like a candy bar, the bonds that hold it together rapidly disintegrate in your stomach.

The individual sugar molecules that were held in place by those bonds make a beeline for your bloodstream, and the rapid spike in blood sugar gives you an intense surge of energy. Unfortunately, it doesn't last long. Because the sugar is rapidly metabolized, the rush it gives you is very short-lived.

In response to the sugar overload in your bloodstream, your pancreas begins to pump out insulin. Insulin is a hormone whose job in life is to attach itself to sugar molecules in the bloodstream and then escort them to various tissues in the body where they can be used for energy.

(continued on page 74)

What About Sugar Substitutes?

If you're worried about eating too much sugar, you may have turned to artificial sweeteners to satisfy your sweet tooth and avoid the caloric consequences. Artificial sweeteners aren't new—cyclamate, marketed as Sweet'N Low, was introduced in 1951. The Food and Drug Administration banned it in 1969, after eight cyclamate-fed laboratory rats developed bladder tumors.

Human beings using cyclamate did not develop bladder tumors, and the decision to ban the product has been cursed and criticized but never rescinded in the United States. After the cyclamate ban, the maker of Sweet'N Low turned to saccharin to fill its little pink packages, but saccharin came under attack next. In 1977, a Canadian scientist reported that male saccharin users had an increased risk of bladder cancer. The FDA toyed with the idea of banning saccharin, but hastily dismissed it after 80,000 outraged dieters and diabetics formally protested. Subsequent studies conceded that saccharin is a minor carcinogen in male rats, but not necessarily in male human beings. Saccharin-containing products are now packaged with a warning label to that effect.

In 1965, a research worker accidentally discovered what would later become aspartame, a product 180 times sweeter than natural sugars. The FDA approved this "safe" sugar substitute in 1981. Marketed as NutraSweet, aspartame didn't take long to become the most popular artificial sweetener in the nation.

Aspartame is made by artificially combining two simple amino acids: aspartic acid and phenylalanine. Individually, both are found in many natural foods, so it would seem safe for human consumption. Although aspartame has been accused of causing nausea, headaches, mood swings, and seizures, testing hasn't uncovered any serious problems in healthy people.

Aspartame does, however, pose a threat to people who lack the enzyme necessary for the breakdown of phenylalanine. This metabolic disorder is known as phenylketonuria, or PKU, and affects about one person in 10,000 in the United States.

The latest sugar substitute to hit the market is the high-intensity artificial sweetener sucralose, sold under the name Splenda. Sucralose is the only noncaloric sweetener made from real sugar. It is produced by selectively adding chlorine atoms to sucrose—simple table sugar—in a patented manufacturing process.

In 1998, the FDA approved sucralose for use in foods and beverages. In 2000, Splenda became available in supermarkets as a tabletop sweetener in two forms: granular and powder. Although Splenda looks and tastes like sugar, it has much less to offer in the way of nutrition. A cup of Splenda Granular has just 96 calories and 24 grams of carbohydrates, compared to the 770 calories and 192 grams of carbohydrates found in each cup of the real stuff. Splenda is about 600 times sweeter than sucrose, making it the sweetest artificial sugar on the market.

The manufacturers of Splenda cite more than two decades of research to support their claims that their product is safe. The results of their studies show that the product isn't toxic or carcinogenic. It has no effect on human reproduction, and it doesn't damage the central nervous system. In fact, the makers of Splenda say that because sucralose is poorly absorbed and rapidly excreted, it doesn't have any effect at all on the human body. But some consumer groups have voiced concern that there isn't enough evidence to support the theory that sucralose will still be safe over the long haul.

While sugar substitutes play an important role in the diets of diabetics trying to maintain control of their blood sugar levels, there is serious doubt as to whether they offer any benefit to folks without the condition. Most of the 163 million Americans who routinely use noncaloric artificial sweeteners are merely supplementing—not replacing—conventional sugars in their diets. The average American adult now consumes well over 100 pounds of sugar each year. As consumption of sugar rises, so does the consumption of sugar substitutes. And in spite of the increasing use of sugar substitutes, more Americans are overweight than ever before. If would seem as though choosing the little

(continued on page 74)

What About Sugar Substitutes?—continued

pink or blue packages over the little white ones would help us stay slim, but there is surprisingly little evidence to support this assumption. Several studies have linked the use of artificial sweeteners to weight *gain*, not weight *loss*. One study showed that women who began drinking diet sodas gained an average of fifteen pounds in the first year.

The reason for the weight gain hasn't been nailed down, but there's good evidence that artificial sweeteners trigger an insulin response in the body, just like real sugar. Insulin's job in life is to escort calories to storage sites in the body. But because there are no calories in artificial sweeteners, insulin levels stay elevated in the bloodstream, stimulating hunger for as long as ninety minutes or more and leading people to eat more than they would if they had just eaten real sugar. If your sweet tooth demands something sweet, it's okay to eat real sugar—just remember to keep track of the amount you eat. Unfortunately, nothing in life is free—not even sugar-free products.

Spurred into action by a big dose of sugar, your pancreas may overshoot the mark and release too much insulin. The excess insulin will soak up more blood sugar than it should, resulting in low blood sugar levels that can leave you feeling weak and shaky. Even worse, it can cause you to feel hungry, which leads you to eat again. This self-defeating cycle can repeat itself dozens of times every day.

Because simple carbohydrates wreak havoc with your insulin, blood sugar, and energy levels, you should keep them to a minimum in your daily diet. No more than 20 percent of your total carbohydrate calories should come from simple carbohydrates.

Complex Carbohydrates

As their name implies, complex carbohydrates are bound together in a complex manner. The bonds that join the individual sugar molecules in a complex carbohydrate food are much more difficult to break apart than the ones in a simple carbohydrate food: they require more digestion in the stomach and intestines. As a result, complex carbohydrates are broken down more slowly in your digestive tract, and the individual sugars that form them are very gradually released into your bloodstream.

The slow, steady release of sugar from complex carbohydrates into your bloodstream doesn't trigger a dramatic insulin response from your pancreas. As the individual sugar molecules are steadily released from your stomach into your blood, you'll notice a gradual, sustained rise in your energy level.

You can think of complex carbohydrate foods as time-released energy foods because they fuel your body and your brain for hours after you eat them. Because carbohydrates of the complex variety are much better for you than those of the simple type, 80 percent of your carbohydrate calories should come from complex carbohydrate foods.

Foods that are rich in complex carbohydrates are not only good for you, they also make you *feel* good. Here are a few reasons why:

Complex carbohydrate foods are high-energy foods

For starters, carbohydrates—especially those of the complex variety—are high-energy, power-packed nutrients. Elite endurance athletes have been onto this fact for years. That's the reason they routinely engage in a practice known as "carbohydrate loading" in preparation for rigorous training and competition.

As you now know, complex carbohydrates are composed of simple sugar molecules that are joined together in a complex configuration. Your digestive system has to work a little to cleave the bonds and separate the individual sugars in complex carbohydrates so that they can be released into your bloodstream and be used for energy. Because the individual sugar molecules are released into the bloodstream in a slow and steady manner, they provide a sustained source of energy.

If you eat a meal that is rich in complex carbohydrates, you'll get a steady supply of energy that will keep your body energized with high-quality fuel for hours. If, on the other hand, you choose to consume a meal that is rich in simple carbohydrates, you'll get an immediate surge of energy, which will soon be followed by a crash. When your energy level hits rock bottom, you may be tempted to refuel your body by eating again, long before it's time for your next meal.

Complex carbohydrate foods are low in fat and calories

Not only are complex carbohydrate foods good sources of energy, they're also naturally low in fat, cholesterol, and calories. If you take a look at people who thrive on high-carbohydrate diets, like natives of Asian countries, you'll notice that most of them are very thin. Diets in Japan and China are typically plant-based and loaded with complex carbohydrates.

Complex carbohydrate foods are low-calorie foods, as long as they're eaten in their natural forms. A simple, unadulterated bowl of oatmeal has about 100 calories, with absolutely no cholesterol or fat. But if you pile butter and sugar on your oatmeal, it's no longer a low-fat, low-calorie food. Now it may have as many as 200 calories and 18 grams of fat. That's no way to treat an innocent little bowl of oatmeal—or your body.

Complex carbohydrates stimulate their own metabolism

Complex carbohydrate foods are naturally low in calories, and the good news is that when you eat them in excess, they're less fattening than high-protein or high-fat foods. If you choose to splurge every now and then, you should make sure that the extra calories that you consume come from complex carbohydrate foods. Why? One reason is that complex carbohydrate foods are more likely to contain certain beneficial nutrients than foods that are high in fat or protein. While you're taking in extra calories, at least you'll be getting some extra vitamins and minerals. Even better, when they're eaten in excess, complex carbohydrates actually stimulate their own metabolism.

Your body uses a great deal of energy in the process of metabolizing complex carbohydrate foods. In terms of their structure, complex carbohydrates bear very little similarity to fat. In order to be converted to body fat, they must first be broken down and then reassembled, a process that is extremely energy-intensive.

If you eat 100 calories more than your body needs to support itself on a given day, and if you get those extra calories from complex carbohydrate foods, your body will use about 25 of those 100 calories in the process of converting the complex carbohydrates to body fat. For every 100 calories of complex carbohydrates that you eat in excess of your daily caloric requirement, only about 75 calories will end up being converted into body fat. The other 25 calories will be burned up in the energy-intensive process of metabolizing the carbohydrates into fat.

If you decide to splurge on a high-protein food, on the other hand, you can't expect to reap the same calorie-saving benefits. Proteins are much more easily converted to body fat than carbohydrates. If you eat 100 calories more than your body needs on a given day, and if you get them from protein-rich foods, your body will use only about 12 of those extra 100 calories in the process of converting the proteins into body fat. You'll end up depositing the remaining 88 calories in your body's fat stores.

Splurging on high-fat foods is even worse because dietary fat bears a very strong structural resemblance to your own body fat. It doesn't take much work at all for your body to convert the fat in a big, juicy hamburger to a type of fat that can be stocked away in body stores. In fact, your body uses only about 3 calories per 100 in the process of converting dietary fat to body fat.

If you decide to indulge and go over your caloric limit on a given day, be sure to choose your bonus calories from complex carbohydrate foods. You'll gain less weight than you would if you ate the same number of extra calories in the form of high-fat or high-protein foods, and you're likely to get a few extra vitamins and minerals to boot.

Complex carbohydrates flip the satiety switch

Carbohydrate-rich foods are important for still another reason. Studies show that carbohydrates are the nutrients primarily responsible for signaling your brain that it's time to stop eating. It was once thought that the amount of food consumed was the most important factor in determining satiety. Scientists speculated that when enough food was eaten to stretch the stomach, nerves in the digestive tract transmitted messages to the satiety center of the brain. The brain, in turn, sent messages to the hand, telling it to stop forking food into the mouth.

While stomach stretching is undoubtedly involved in creating feelings of satiety to some degree, it's not the most important factor at work. If it were, simply drinking a couple of glasses of water would be enough to stretch your stomach and satisfy your hunger.

More recently, scientists have discovered that the satiety signal in your brain is activated when complex carbohydrates are consumed. A meal rich in complex carbohydrates not only stretches your stomach; it sends messages to your central nervous system that you've had enough to eat, and it's time to stop.

Your body adjusts your appetite and down-regulates your eating in response to the number of complex carbohydrates present in the foods that you eat. The higher the complex carbohydrate content of your meal, the more satisfaction you'll derive from eating it, and the sooner your brain will let you know that you've had quite enough, thank you.

With this in mind, you can see why getting an adequate amount of complex carbohydrates in your diet is so important. Roughly half of the calories in each meal or snack you eat should come from carbohydrates, and you have to make sure that the carbohydrate foods that you choose are those made up of complex carbohydrates, not simple ones. Appetite signals arising from simple carbohydrate foods, such as cakes, cookies, and candy, are very different from those that arise from complex carbohydrates. Simple carbohydrates don't suppress your appetite at all; in fact, they may even stimulate your hunger.

Simple carbohydrates are easily converted to sugar in your body. Because we derive such intense pleasure from eating them, humans have an innate preference for sweet foods. We like sugar so much that when we eat it, our appetite suppression signals tend to be blatantly ignored or overridden. Since sugar doesn't flip the satiety switch in the brain, eating too many simple carbohydrate foods on a regular basis can lead to overeating, which in turn leads to weight gain.

By eliminating most simple carbohydrate foods from your diet and replacing them with complex carbohydrate foods, you'll be the recipient of two very important benefits. First, your diet will immediately be lower in calories. In spite of consuming fewer calories, you'll feel more satisfied after eating, and you'll be less vulnerable to the temptation of snacking between meals. You'll also find that your energy levels will be dramatically higher, and they'll stay that way much longer after eating. When you eat foods that give you more energy and less hunger, you'll find that weight loss will be much easier than you imagined possible.

Complex carbohydrates are rich in fiber

Another benefit of eating complex carbohydrate foods is that they are naturally loaded with fiber. Fiber forms the structural framework of plants, and human beings lack the enzyme necessary to digest it. As a result, fiber travels through your gastrointestinal tract pretty much unchanged, and that's what makes it so useful.

Fiber helps ward off constipation by attracting water in the digestive tract to help create softer stools. By virtue of its bulk, fiber dilutes the concentration of cancer-causing agents in the colon. It binds to carcinogens and disarms them before they can do any major damage. And because fiber speeds the intestinal contents toward their ultimate destination, carcinogens spend less time in the colon and have less opportunity to work their cancer-causing mischief.

A high-fiber diet has also been shown to protect your heart by lowering cholesterol levels. Fiber is thought to reduce blood cholesterol levels in a couple of different ways. Friendly bacteria in your colon convert fiber to products that eventually block the formation of cholesterol. Fiber also binds with formed cholesterol, preventing it from being absorbed into your bloodstream. Eating a high-fiber diet allows you to lose more cholesterol in your stool and deposit less of it on your artery walls.

Foods rich in fiber can help you lose weight. They're bulky, filling, and low in calories. They take longer to eat because they require some serious chewing, and this property dramatically increases their satiety value. People who consume high-fiber diets are typically thinner than those whose diets are low in fiber.

Research has shown that eating high-fiber meals triggers the release of cholecystokinin in the body, a substance that is also released when fatty meals are consumed. Elevated levels of cholecystokinin are associated with feelings of satiety, and the consumption of fiber not only stimulates its release, it also prolongs its presence in the bloodstream after eating. Fiber

Add Fiber to Your Diet

Choose high-fiber cereals:

General Mills Fiber One, with 13 grams of fiber per serving

Kellogg's All-Bran, with 10 grams of fiber per serving

Kellogg's Raisin Bran, with 8 grams of fiber per serving

Post 100% Bran Flakes, with 5 grams of fiber per serving

Eat more of the following foods:

Bran muffins

All-bran cereals

Multigrain cereals, cooked or dry

Whole-wheat bread

Oatmeal

Popcorn

Cooked beans

Choose fruits and vegetables that are fiber-rich:

Apples	Garbanzo beans (chickpeas)
Berries	Green peas
Broccoli	Kidney beans
Brussels sprouts	Lima beans
Carrots	Oranges
Cauliflower	Pears
Figs	Prunes

pushes food through the digestive system at a steady clip, allowing less time for calories to be absorbed into your bloodstream.

While most foods that are rich in complex carbohydrates are high in fiber, many simple carbohydrate foods, like fruits and vegetables, are also loaded with roughage. Until recently, there hasn't been a formal dietary fiber recommendation for kids. Nutrition experts at the Institute for Cancer Prevention now use the "Age Plus Five" rule as a guideline for fiber consumption among children. The current recommendation for dietary fiber for children ages three to eighteen is 1 gram for each year of age, plus 5 grams. For an eight-year-old child, the recommended amount is 8 plus 5 grams, for a total of 12 grams of fiber a day. Adults are advised to aim for 20 to 35 grams a day, an amount that is more than double what most Americans take in. You don't have to eat a bale of hay to get your fiber, but it does take a little effort. Eating the recommended five servings of fruits and vegetables and six servings of whole-grain foods, cereals, and legumes each day will help you reach your goal. You can also increase your daily fiber consumption by adding whole-bran products to recipes ranging from pancakes to meatloaf.

Complex carbohydrates stimulate neurotransmitter production

Complex carbohydrate foods play another vital role in your diet. They stimulate your body's production of a neurotransmitter called serotonin and a hormone called norepinephrine. Norepinephrine is structurally similar to adrenaline, and like adrenaline, it increases your energy levels. Even better, it boosts your body's metabolic rate. The higher your metabolic rate, the more calories you burn, even while you're at rest.

The brain chemical serotonin has been shown to have several important roles in the human body. It is known to have a calming effect and to help ward off depression. People who are severely depressed have lower blood levels of serotonin than happier folk.

Several prescription antidepressant drugs work to reduce anxiety and depression by increasing levels of the neurotransmitter serotonin in the central nervous system. If you've ever found yourself eating in response to anxiety, depression, or stress, you may have noticed that the foods you crave are rich in carbohydrates. This is your body's built-in mechanism to increase serotonin levels in your brain.

Not only is Serotonin an important mood stabilizer, it's also an effective appetite regulator. Many prescription appetite-suppressant drugs work by increasing levels of serotonin in the central nervous system.

You can get many of the benefits that these medicines have to offer simply by boosting your daily intake of complex carbohydrates. A diet that is rich in complex carbohydrates not only makes you feel good physically, it also increases your level of emotional well-being. Both make weight loss much easier to achieve and maintain.

Complex carbohydrate foods are a vital part of a well-balanced diet. They're high-fiber foods that are naturally low in fat, calories, and cholesterol, and they're typically excellent sources of beneficial vitamins and minerals. They help suppress your appetite and boost your energy levels, even while you're cutting back on calories. Even better, foods that are rich in complex carbohydrates are readily available, inexpensive, and easy to prepare.

Carbohydrate Requirements

Calories from carbohydrate foods contribute half of your daily caloric intake in the G-Factor Program. If you consume 2,000 calories a day, 1,000 of these calories should come from carbohydrate foods. Of these 1,000 carbohydrate calories, 80 percent, or 800 calories, should come from complex carbohydrate sources, and no more than 20 percent, or 200 calories, should come from simple carbohydrate sources.

Both simple and complex carbohydrates have 4 calories per gram. If your G-Factor Program calls for 1,000 carbohydrate calories a day, you'll be eating a total of 250 grams of carbohydrates. Eighty percent, or 200 grams, should come from complex carbohydrate foods, while 20 percent, or 50 grams, should come from simple carbohydrate foods.

2. Protein

Even when you're eating all the carbohydrates that your body needs, there's still plenty of room left in your diet for protein. Proteins, an important part of the G-Factor Program, are vital to your good health. No matter what kind of shape you're in, your body requires as much protein as any world-class athlete, and your protein requirements generally don't slack off as you age.

Protein is an important part of a well-balanced diet for several reasons. For starters, protein makes up about a fifth of your total body weight. Most of it is stored in your muscles, but it is also an important component of your bones, cartilage, skin, organs, and even body fluids. Proteins are used to help carry out important biochemical reactions throughout your body.

Your immune system is made up entirely of proteins. Your body depends on replacement proteins in your diet to keep your defense systems functioning properly, so that you're able to fend off infections and diseases.

In your diet, protein is a source of long-lasting energy. You should include some high-quality protein foods at every meal, especially breakfast. Together, protein and complex carbohydrate foods effectively stave off hunger until it's time for your next snack or meal.

If you're a meat eater, getting enough protein in your daily diet probably isn't a problem for you. Most Americans eat more than twice the amount of protein they need on a daily basis. At the same time, however, they're shortchanging themselves on complex carbohydrates, eating less than half the recommended daily amount. A diet that is long on protein and short on complex carbohydrates is not only unbalanced, it's unhealthy.

Protein Sources

Protein-rich foods aren't hard to find, but sometimes healthy, low-fat sources of protein can seem a little scarce or expensive at the very least. Animal products of all types are excellent sources of protein, but on the downside, many of them are loaded with fat, cholesterol, and calories.

Lean meats and low-fat dairy products—including lean beef, skinless chicken, fish, skim milk, and fat-free cheese—are good sources of animal protein. In the produce department, dried beans, peas, and other legumes are excellent sources. Protein can be found in corn, rice, and pasta, as well. In spite of their bad reputation, nuts and eggs are excellent sources of high-quality protein.

The Problem with High-Protein Diets

Protein is a vital part of your healthy diet, but you don't want to go overboard. You certainly don't want to go on one of those high-protein fad diets. Many overweight adults and adolescents have tried these diets, and some actually managed to lose weight—at least temporarily. But success has its price; high-protein diets can take a serious toll on your health.

The founders of the high-protein diets claim that they've discovered the "real" secret to weight loss. It's the carbohydrates in our diets that are making us fat, they say. Foods that we once thought were good—like fruits and veggies, cereal and pasta—are now bad. The protein pushers say that carbohydrate foods stimulate the production of insulin (true), and that high insulin levels make you fat (false). That's where the protein pushers twist the facts: high insulin levels don't make you overweight—being over-weight causes you to have high insulin levels.

The protein peddlers have a simple solution, based on this misinformation. If you would only cut your carbohydrate intake, you could lower your insulin levels, and every ounce of unsightly blubber on your body would effortlessly evaporate.

Some high-protein diets call for a measly 20 to 30 grams of carbohydrates a day. This type of nutritional blasphemy is enough to make most doctors and nutrition experts gnash their teeth and tear their hair out. To keep your carbohydrate consumption to a bare minimum, you're advised to eat mostly protein and fat. You're given the go-ahead to chow down on cheese, bacon, butter, and big juicy steaks. What a great diet!

But the benefits of the high-protein diets come to a screeching halt right after your taste buds. When you drastically lower your carbohydrate intake, blood sugar becomes scarce. Your body thinks it's starving, and it activates a rescue mode, called ketosis. In this precarious metabolic state, your body is forced to burn some of its own fat to produce the energy it needs to survive.

The fat-burning part sounds great, but there are a few problems associated with ketosis, ranging from annoying to life-threatening. Ketosis can alter the concentration of electrolytes in your blood, leaving you shaky and dizzy. You may find yourself too sick or weak to eat—a bonus benefit of the diet.

Ketosis also taints your breath, perspiration, and urine with a vile odor. Some people liken it to the stench of rotten apples; others compare it to sewer gas. Since the odor emanates from your lungs and even your very pores, there's no disguising it with breath mints or perfumes. Clipping an air freshener onto your clothing might be most helpful.

If you've got a problem with diarrhea, you're going to love this diet—your bowels may lock up for days on end. Eating nothing but meat and cheese is going to leave you with a serious fiber shortage. But don't bother trying to take a laxative, because a couple of tablespoons of Metamucil can blow your carbohydrate allowance for the day.

As long as you're losing weight, you might as well lose some of that extra bone mass you've been packing around. A high-protein diet steals calcium from your bones and reroutes it directly to your toilet bowl, via your urine. Over the long haul, it can increase your risk for bone fractures and osteoporosis. To be on the safe side, you'll need to take a supplement while you're dieting. Since you're already constipated from the lack of fiber, you shouldn't even notice the effects of the calcium.

If you're prone to develop gout, now is an excellent time for a flare-up. High-protein foods are notorious for triggering attacks. Last but not least, you'll just have to ignore the decades of hard scientific evidence linking diets high in fat and protein with an increased risk for heart disease and cancer. Besides, who cares if you knock a few years off your life expectancy? At least you'll leave a thin corpse, and maybe you can be buried in a Spandex bodysuit and a formfitting casket.

Protein Requirements

A diet too rich in protein is definitely bad for you, but an adequate amount is vital to your good health. Calories from protein foods make up 30 percent of the G-Factor Program. If, for example, you need 2,000 calories a day, 600 of those calories should come from protein-rich foods. Like carbohydrates, proteins have 4 calories per gram, so a well-balanced diet consisting of 2,000 calories a day includes about 112 grams of protein.

3. Fat

Dietary fat has gotten a bad rap in recent years. With the increasing popularity of low-fat and no-fat diets, Americans have developed an unhealthy degree of fat phobia.

It's true that too much fat in the diet contributes to a thousand ills, like obesity, high cholesterol levels, heart disease, and some types of cancer, but some fat in your diet is not only beneficial, it's absolutely essential. Too little fat in the diet can be dangerous for adults, and even more so for growing kids.

Fat is found in every cell in the human body. It stores energy, keeps your skin soft and supple, and cushions and protects your internal organs. Most importantly, fat stores and circulates the fat-soluble vitamins A, D, E, and K in your body. Because fat-free foods don't contain fat-soluble vitamins, a diet that is devoid of fat is nutritionally incomplete and potentially harmful. And if you think that vitamin supplements can satisfy your daily requirements for vitamis A, D, E, and K, think again: Without fat, these vitamins cannot be properly metabolized by your body.

Fat Sources

You probably don't need any help pegging the fat-rich foods in your diet. Any food that leaves a greasy spot in its wake is a good source of dietary fat. Butters, oils, most fast foods, and animal products, such as meat and dairy foods, are all good sources of dietary fat.

Many high-protein and carbohydrate-rich foods are also high in hidden fat, so be sure to check the nutrition labels. Fatty foods should be eaten with a big dose of moderation, but it's not necessary to eliminate them completely from your diet.

Fat requirements

Most experts agree that under no circumstances should fat be reduced for children under the age of two years. Restricting or limiting fat intake for infants younger than twenty-four months can interfere with their growth and development.

For older children and adults following the G-Force Program, 20 percent of the daily caloric intake will come from fat. Children, teens, and adults who are healthy and of normal weight or underweight may safely consume as much as 30 percent of their total daily caloric intake in the form of fat.

Getting enough fat in the diet isn't a problem for most folks. Typical Americans consume more than twice the amount they need on a daily basis. Following the G-Factor Program, a diet that consists of 2,000 calories a day will include only 400 calories from fat. Unlike carbohydrates and proteins, which have just 4 calories per gram, fat has a whopping 9 calories per gram. That's what makes it so fattening. If you consume 400 calories of fat each day, you'll be getting around 44 grams of fat.

While it's important to be aware of the amount of fat that makes its way into your family's diet, it's just as important to know what kinds of fat you're consuming. High-quality fats help promote good health and ward off a slew of ailments and illnesses. There are three main types of dietary fat: *polyunsaturated*, *monounsaturated*, and *saturated*. Of these, fats of the polyunsaturated variety are considered to be the most beneficial.

Saturated fats are the nutritional bad guys. They usually exist in a solid form at room temperature, and they're derived primarily from animal sources, like meats and dairy products. Some plant oils, including palm oil and coconut oil, are also saturated, and they're just as bad for you as animal fats. Saturated fats are often tucked away in cookies, cakes, chocolate, and other junk foods. Eating too many saturated fats can drive up your cholesterol levels, an event that can lead to blocked arteries and, eventually, heart disease. After the age of two years, children, like adults, should limit their saturated fats to no more than 5 to 10 percent of their daily calories.

Polyunsaturated fats are the dietary good guys. They usually exist in a liquid state at room temperature, and they're found in many plant oils, like sunflower, safflower, soybean, and sesame seed oils. These friendly fats are also found in cold-water fish, including tuna, halibut, sardines, and salmon.

Polyunsaturated oils contain health-promoting substances called essential fatty acids, or EFAs. Because your body isn't capable of manufacturing these substances, you have to consume them in your diet. If you're like most folks, you probably don't get enough EFAs for optimum health. An estimated 80 percent of Americans consume diets that are deficient in essential fatty acids. Highly processed convenience foods, which make up a large part of the typical U.S. diet, are often deliberately stripped of many EFAs to prolong their shelf life.

Diets that are lacking in EFAs can promote or worsen many medical maladies, including diabetes, arthritis, and skin disorders such as psoriasis and eczema. Inadequate consumption of these health-promoting substances can aggravate the symptoms of premenstrual syndrome and emotional disorders.

Recent research suggests that diets rich in EFAs may help strengthen bones and play an important role in the prevention of osteoporosis. Essential fatty acids have been shown to increase calcium absorption from the intestines, while reducing excretion of the mineral through the urinary tract.

The essential fatty acids found in fish oils may help reduce your risk of cancer. This protective effect was first observed in Greenland Eskimos, who thrive on fish-based diets and have significantly lower rates of certain types of cancer than their American counterparts.

Essential fatty acids play an important role in pregnancy, promoting normal growth of tissues and organs in the developing fetus. Maternal diets that are deficient in EFAs have been linked to low birth weights and poorly developed central nervous systems in newborns.

While diets high in cholesterol and saturated fats are known to con-tribute to heart disease, diets rich in EFAs have been shown to reduce the risk. They seem to help prevent blood clots in the heart's arteries, decrease inflammation in blood vessel walls, and support a regular heart rhythm. In spite of their nutritional benefits, it's still a good idea to limit your intake of polyunsaturated fats to no more then 8 to 10 percent of your total daily caloric intake.

Monounsaturated fats also fall into the category of friendly fats. They help lower total cholesterol levels as well as low-density lipoproteins in the blood. Low-density lipoproteins are the "bad" type of cholesterol that can accumulate in blood vessels and contribute to hardening of the arteries and heart disease. Monounsaturated fats are found in olive oil, peanuts, avo-cados, some nuts, and canola oil. They should be limited to about 10 per-cent of your daily caloric intake.

If you're trying to reduce your family's fat consumption, your best bet is to avoid fast food, processed food, and junk food. But don't let fat phobia cause you and your family to miss out on the friendly fats that are vital to good health.

Fake Fat: Olestra

It sounds almost too good to be true—snacking on junk food can be a totally fat-free experience. The miracle substance that renders snack foods fat-free is olestra, marketed under the trade name Olean. Invented over thirty years ago, the compound has been subjected to an ongoing series of rigorous laboratory, animal, and human safety testing. In January 1996, the product finally gained the official thumbs-up from the U.S. Food and Drug Administration.

Olestra is a fat-replacement product made by combining simple sugars with vegetable oil. The fat and sugars in the faux fat are locked together in a unique combination that makes the resulting molecules much larger than ordinary fat molecules. The human digestive system is totally incapable of breaking them down, and as a result, they never make it to those pesky little fat cells in other body parts.

The upside to this wonder substance is that it is completely fat free and devoid of calories. Using it to replace the regular fat in snack foods reduces the calories per serving from 150 calories to just 70, saving you about 80 calories every time you snack. If you eat a serving of chips every day, replacing your high-fat brand with an olestra-containing brand will net you a weight loss of about a pound and a half every month. Over the course of a year, you're looking at lightening your load by a grand total of eighteen pounds, a weight loss that many folks could use.

And while you're dodging some extra calories, you won't be missing out on any flavor. Like regular fat, olestra adds a rich taste and smooth texture to foods. Most people agree that snacks made with olestra are just as tasty as the real thing. Unless you're a card-carrying junk food connoisseur, you probably won't be able to tell the difference.

But for some folks, there's a teeny-tiny downside to olestra consumption. Since the fake fat isn't absorbed, it remains in the digestive tract. While it's there, it can cause a few problems, like intestinal cramping, gas, loose stools, and for a select few, the unthinkable—fecal urgency.

A single serving of olestra-containing chips, popcorn, or crackers doesn't cause side effects in most people. But if you tend to get carried away with your snacking, consider yourself warned. Multiple servings may lead to gastrointestinal distress. The more olestra you consume, the more likely you are to serve time in solitary confinement in the smallest room in your house.

Olestra isn't alone in its ability to send you scurrying in search of a bathroom. Other products, like mineral oil, some artificial sweeteners, and the fibrous portions of plants, travel through your innards undigested, leading to similar problems. The difference lies in your ability to exercise portion control. While you probably wouldn't dream of wolfing down an entire box of raisin bran in one sitting, you may have absolutely no qualms about munching your way through a bag of fat-free chips.

Some experts aren't as concerned about the gastrointestinal effects of olestra as they are about the nutritional implications. There is some concern that the fat-soluble vitamins A, D, E, and K may be whisked out of the human digestive tract on the coattails of the olestra. With this in mind, the federal government now requires olestra-containing products to be fortified with these vitamins. It's probably not a good idea to allow children to eat products made with olestra on a regular basis. Numerous studies based on millions of servings consumed have demonstrated that olestra is safe for human consumption, with gastrointestinal woes being the most serious side effect.

Snack foods made with olestra are slightly more expensive than regular brands, but if spending a few extra cents saves you a few extra pounds, they're well worth the price.

Putting the G-Factor Program to Work

Now that you know the basics of the G-Factor Program, it's time to apply them to your family's diet. For toddlers and preschoolers, simply providing a well-balanced diet with a variety of selections from the five food groups is usually all it takes to prevent weight problems. For most school-age children, reducing the daily intake by just 250 calories will result in the loss of about half a pound per week, or two pounds per month. A loss of two pounds a month won't jeopardize your child's health, growth, or development, and the slow, steady weight loss is more likely to be permanent than rapid weight loss. If you and your child remind yourselves that there are twelve months in the year, you'll probably agree that losing a couple of pounds a month can bring about dramatic results.

Unlike your younger kids, you and your older children will benefit from a little more guidance and structure. For adults and children ages sixteen and up, the G-Factor Program Worksheet will make balancing the diet easier.

Before filling out the worksheet, you'll need identify your goal weight and determine how many total calories should be consumed each day in order to reach it. Most moderately active adults need roughly 11 calories each day to support each pound of their body weight. If, for example, you weigh 150 pounds, you'll need to eat about 1,650 calories every day to maintain that weight, because 150 x 11 is 1,650.

What if your goal weight is 150 pounds, but you currently weigh 200 pounds? If you weigh 200 pounds right now, your daily diet probably consists of around 2,200 calories, because 200 x 11 is equal to 2,200, and it takes about 2,200 calories a day to support 200 pounds of body weight for a reasonably active person.

If you want to weigh 150 pounds, you have to start eating like a 150-pound person. If you feed only 150 pounds of your body, those unwanted 50 pounds will eventually get lost. By feeding your 200-pound body 1,650 calories a day instead of 2,200 calories a day, you'll be cutting your intake by 550 calories, which is enough to net you a weight loss of a little more than a pound a week. As you continue to slim down, your weight loss will gradually slow, but eventually, you will reach your goal weight of 150 pounds. It sounds too simple to be true, but it works.

Now you know the G-Factors for carbohydrate, protein, and fat that you'll need to meet to lose weight and then maintain your ideal weight. The good news is that you'll be eating a nutritious, well-balanced diet in the process.

Decoding Nutrition Labels

Balancing your G-Factors is going to take a little effort at first, because you might not be familiar with the nutrient contents of many foods. Fortunately, all packaged foods in the United States now come with a handy nutrition label attached.

In the not too distant past, food labels barely even identified what was actually inside a box or bag. Folks pretty much just had to try the food and hope for the best. But during the twentieth century, the U.S. Food and Drug Administration got involved in the regulation of food labeling, and the organization created a lot of rules in the process. In 1990, the Nutrition Labeling and Education Act was born, and together, the Food and Drug Administration and the U.S. Department of Agriculture implemented changes that made food labels easier for consumers to understand. Launched in 1994, the "Nutrition Facts" labels included five major changes.

For starters, the nutrition information is printed in a larger and more legible type so that you don't have to use a magnifying glass with the power of the Hubble Telescope to make out the words. A new column of informa-

The G-Factor Program Worksheet

Determining the nutrient needs for yourself and your older children is as easy as filling in the blanks on the G-Factor Program Worksheet. Let's get started!

Daily Caloric Needs

Goal weight _____ x 11 = Daily caloric intake
Your daily caloric intake is the number of calories your body needs to support itself at your goal weight.
_____ Daily caloric intake

Daily Nutrient Needs

A healthy, well-balanced diet consists of 50 percent carbohydrates, 30 percent protein, and 20 percent fat.

Since 50 percent of your daily calories should come from carbohydrate foods, multiply your daily caloric intake by .50 to determine the total number of carbohydrate calories you should eat every day:
_____ Carbohydrate calories

Since there are 4 calories in each gram of carbohydrate, divide this number by 4 to get the total number of carbohydrate grams you should eat each day:
_____ G-Factor for carbohydrates

tion, titled "% Daily Value," tells you how the food at hand fits into a well-balanced diet. The label must also include information about saturated fat, cholesterol, fiber, vitamins, and minerals.

Another important change is that serving sizes listed are now closer to the amounts that real people actually eat. In the past, manufacturers could get away with passing a single cookie off as two or three servings, making

---

Proteins make up 30 percent of the G-Factor Program. Multiply your daily caloric intake by 30 to determine the number of protein calories you should eat every day:

_____Protein calories

Since there are 4 calories in each gram of protein, divide this number by 4 to get the total number of protein grams you should eat each day:

_____G-Factor for protein

Fat makes up 20 percent of the G-Factor Program. Multiply your daily caloric intake by .20 to determine the number of fat calories you should eat every day:

_____Fat calories

Each gram of fat has 9 calories, so divide this number by 9 to get the number of fat grams you should eat every day:

_____G-Factor for fat

From here on, the only numbers you'll need to remember are your G-Factors for carbohydrates, protein, and fat. If you match your G-Factors on a daily basis, everything else will take care of itself. You'll be eating a healthy diet, and you'll be losing weight! Write those numbers here:

_____G-Factor for carbohydrate

_____G-Factor for protein

_____G-Factor for fat

it appear to have less fat, sugar, and calories, but these types of tricks no longer fly. Health claims made by food manufacturers, like "light" or "low fat," must now meet strict government definitions so that they are not only accurate but also consistent from one food to another.

To make wise choices about the foods that you eat, it's important to understand the various parts of the nutrition label.

Serving Size. At the top of each food label, you'll find a serving size amount. The serving size, the amount of the food you must eat to obtain all the nutrients listed, is based on the amount that people generally eat, according to standards set by the Food and Drug Administration. The serving size listed may not be the recommended amount, but it is the typical amount consumed. Remember to multiply the fat, calories, and other nutrients listed by the number of servings you eat.

Calories. The calorie is a standard unit that measures the amount of energy provided to your body by food. On the food label, the number listed tells you how many calories you'll get in a single serving. Although daily caloric requirements vary from person to person, food labels are based on a diet of 2000 calories per day.

Calories from Fat. This figure gives you the number of calories in a serving that are provided by fat, making it easier for you to keep track of the fat in your daily diet.

Percent Daily Values. The percent daily values are based on a 2000-calorie-per-day diet. The numbers listed in the right-hand column are given in percentages, allowing you to determine the amount of nutrients you'll get from a single serving. You'll want to get 100 percent of these nutrients over the course of the day. If a percent daily value for calcium in a particular food is listed as 25 percent, you'll know that you've met 25 percent of your daily goal for calcium, and you'll need to get another 75 percent from other food sources. Percent daily values make it easier to determine whether a food is a good source or a poor source of certain nutrients. If a food has 5 percent or less of a given nutrient, it is considered to be low in that nutrient. If the percent daily value of a given nutrient is between 10 and 19 percent, it is considered to be a good source, and if it offers more than 20 percent, it is a rich source of the given nutrient.

Total Fat. This number tells you how much fat you'll get from a single serving of food. The number is typically given in grams.

Saturated Fat. This number gives you the number of grams of saturated fat you'll get from a single serving of food. Remember, saturated fats are the dietary bad guys. They're the ones that can lead to high cholesterol levels and hardening of the arteries, increasing the risk for heart disease and strokes.

Unsaturated Fat. This figure gives you the number of grams of unsaturated fat, the heart-friendly type of fat. Because unsaturated fats don't elevate cholesterol levels, they don't contribute to heart disease when eaten in moderation.

Cholesterol. The amount of cholesterol provided by a single serving of food is listed under the fat information and is given in terms of milligrams. Cholesterol is a fat-like substance that serves as a building block for vitamin D and hormones. Too much dietary cholesterol can lead to high cholesterol levels in the bloodstream, contributing to heart disease and strokes in later life.

Sodium. The amount of sodium (a component of salt) in a single serving of food is listed in units of milligrams. If you're on a sodium-restricted diet, you'll want to pay close attention to this number.

Total Carbohydrate. This number, given in grams, represents the combined total of several types of carbohydrates, including dietary fiber, sugars, and other carbohydrates.

Dietary Fiber. Found under total carbohydrates, dietary fiber is listed in grams.

Sugars. Sugars are found in most foods, especially junk foods. Calories from sugar are typically empty calories, containing few beneficial nutrients.

Vitamin A. Vitamin A is usually the first in a long list of vitamins and minerals on the food label. The amount of vitamin A, as well as other important vitamins and minerals in a single serving of food, is usually listed as a percent daily value. Vitamin A is important for good eyesight and to maintain healthy skin. Dark green, leafy vegetables and orange vegetables, such as carrots and squash, are rich sources of vitamin A.

Vitamin C. This vitamin, found mainly in citrus fruits, is used by the body to heal wounds and fight infection.

Calcium. This mineral is important for healthy bones and teeth and is found primarily in dairy products. It takes three to four cups of dairy products to meet daily calcium needs.

Iron. Iron is used by the body in the production of healthy red blood cells, which carry oxygen throughout the body. Red meat is the best source, but the mineral is also found in milk, iron-fortified cereals, raisins, and dark green, leafy vegetables.

Calories per Gram. This information is printed on food labels for reference, to remind you that there are 9 calories in each gram of fat, and 4 calories in each gram of carbohydrate and protein.

If you take a look at the sample nutrition label for a breakfast cereal, you'll find all the information you need to determine the amounts of carbohydrates, protein, and fat contained in the cereal. Because cereal is typically consumed with milk, nutrition information is also given for the combination of one cup of cereal combined with a half cup of skim milk. According to this label, a single serving size is one cup of cereal, and this amount of food contains 23 grams of carbohydrates, 6 grams of protein, and 0 grams of fat.

Determining the nutrient content of the food that you eat is easy when it comes packaged with a nutrition label. But it's not quite as simple to figure out the nutrient content of the foods that you prepare from scratch or those that you eat in restaurants. For these types of foods, you can consult books or web sites with listings of nutrition information for almost every food available.

You won't have to consult nutrition labels every time you open your mouth to eat, but it's important to do it initially. Before long, you'll get a feel for the nutrient values of different foods, and eating a well-balanced diet will come naturally.

This will give you a good start toward designing your G-Factor Program. Now it's time to put it all together in a daily diet plan. Remember, you don't have to limit yourself to certain foods every day. You just have to make wise choices so that at the end of every day, your actual nutrient totals match your G-Factors for carbohydrates, proteins, and fats.

Nutrition Facts

Serving Size   1 cup (31 g/1.1 oz.)
Servings per Package   About 11

Amount Per Serving	Cereal	Cereal with ½ cup skim milk
Calories	110	150
Calories from fat	0	0

	% Daily Value **	
Total Fat 0 g*	0%	0%
Saturated Fat 0 g	0%	0%
Cholesterol 0 mg	0%	0%
Sodium 220 mg	9%	12%
Potassium 60 mg	2%	7%
Total Carbohydrate 23 g	8%	10%
Dietary Fiber 1 g	4%	4%
Sugars 4 g		
Other Carbohydrate 18 g		
Protein 6 g		
Vitamin A	15%	20%
Vitamin C	35%	35%
Calcium	0%	15%
Iron	45%	45%
Vitamin E	35%	35%
Thiamin	35%	40%
Riboflavin	35%	45%
Niacin	35%	35%
Vitamin B1	35%	35%
Folate	35%	35%
Vitamin B12	35%	45%
Phosphorus	6%	20%
Magnesium	4%	8%
Zinc	6%	8%
Selenium	10%	10%

* Amount in cereal. One half cup of skim milk contributes an additional 65 mg sodium, 6 g total carbohydrate (6 g sugars), and 4 g protein.

**Percent daily values are based on a 2,000 calorie diet. Your daily values may be higher or lower depending on your calorie needs.

Calories		2,000	2,500
Total Fat	Less than	65 g	80 g
Sat. Fat	Less than	20 g	25 g
Cholesterol	Less than	300 mg	300 mg
Sodium	Less than	2,400 mg	2,400 mg
Potassium		3,500 mg	3,500 mg
Total Carbohydrate		300 mg	375 mg
Dietary Fiber		25 g	30 g

Calories per gram: Fat 9 * Carbohydrate 4 * Protein 4

G-Factors for Favorite Foods

To familiarize yourself with the nutrient content of the foods you normally eat, try this simple exercise. List the foods that you enjoy eating for breakfast, consult the nutrition labels on their packages to learn about the nutrients they provide, and record their nutrient contents. Then do the same for your favorite lunch, snack, and dinner foods.

	Food	Carbohydrate	Protein	Fat
Breakfast Foods				
Lunch Foods				
Snack Foods				
Dinner Foods				
Totals				

Daily G-Factor Nutrient Log

If you want to see how close your way of eating comes to a well-balanced diet, try listing everything you ate yesterday, along with the numbers of carbohydrate, protein, and fat grams your meals and snacks provided.

	Food	Carbohydrate	Protein	Fat
Breakfast Foods				
Lunch Foods				
Snack Foods				
Dinner Foods				
Totals				

Now it's time for the acid test—compare yesterday's totals with the recommended G-Factors from your Nutrition Worksheet. How close did you come to eating a balanced diet?

Chapter 6

Beyond Pop-Tarts

Your own mother always told you to eat a good breakfast, and you have probably tried to encourage your kids to do the same. Moms are offering good advice, but not everyone is listening. A third of American kids and adults skip breakfast on a regular basis.

Breakfast Skippers Beware

You may not realize it, but skipping the morning meal throws a huge monkey wrench into your body's internal machinery every single time you do it. The body part most affected is your brain. The human brain relies almost exclusively on blood sugar, or glucose, to fuel its everyday activities. As its primary source of energy, your brain needs glucose as much as it needs oxygen to function properly and even survive. But there's one major hitch in the system: your brain is a lean, mean thinking machine, and it's not equipped with storage tanks for glucose.

With no means of storage, your brain is forced to rely on your bloodstream to deliver the glucose it must have on a minute-to-minute basis. Glucose is easily obtained from carbohydrate-rich foods, like fruits, vegetables, cereal and bread. As long as you eat every five or six hours, there's plenty of easily accessible glucose in the bloodstream, and your brain operates optimally on all cylinders.

Sleeping creates a problem. When you eat your last meal of the day, some of the nutrients from the food roam around in your bloodstream, and some are stored. The nutrients in the bloodstream are used to meet your immediate and short-tem energy needs, and the stored energy is saved for later. The human body is capable of tucking away energy in one of three forms: fat, protein, and a substance called glycogen. Glycogen is simply a chain of glucose molecules that is stored in your liver. The phase of fueling up is called the anabolic, or building, phase, and the hormone that makes it possible is insulin.

If you eat your last meal of the day at around six o'clock, your stomach is happy, and your brain is happy. Over the next six to eight hours, your brain will use up most of the glucose that is circulating freely in your bloodstream, and around midnight, it will start signaling for more. Because you're asleep, you won't be able to respond to this signal by grabbing a bite to eat. But that's okay, because Mother Nature worked out this little glitch ahead of time. The glucose that was stored in your liver as glycogen during the anabolic phase is simply released into your bloodstream. With a fresh supply of fuel, your brain is happy again, but it's only a temporary fix. Your liver is able to store only small amounts of glycogen, just enough to supply your brain with glucose for about eight to ten hours. If you're under a lot of stress or suffering from an illness, the protective period is even shorter.

When your alarm clock blasts you out of bed the next morning, you hit the ground running for the six o'clock scramble. As you tear through the house rousing kids, searching for lost shoes, and preparing for the mad dash to school and work, breakfast may be the very last thing on your mind. But if you don't take time to break the fast, you're headed for trouble. Unbeknownst to you, your liver is spitting out the last of its stored glycogen. Glucose levels in your bloodstream are extremely low, and your brain is now running on fumes.

Deprived of the fuel it must have to operate, your brain starts to sputter. This may cause you to develop a headache or start to feel dizzy. Your concentration and coordination are shot. Your IQ drops about 50 points or so, and your short-term memory is seriously impaired. Even as it's faltering, your brain is activating emergency procedures in your body. It directs your liver to start making glucose from scratch. The liver is capable of manufacturing glucose in a crunch, but it needs several ingredients first.

One of the key ingredients necessary for the de novo production of glucose is supplied by muscle protein. The liver also needs a pinch of a substance called glycerol, which is supplied by fat cells in your body. In the process of making glucose from scratch, very little fat is burned, but a substantial amount of muscle tissue is sacrificed.

The breakdown of muscle tissue to form glucose is known as the catabolic, or breakdown, phase. One of the hormones that make this process possible is adrenaline. Adrenaline sets the breakdown process in motion, but it also has several rather unpleasant side effects. As one of the primary "fight or flight" hormones, adrenaline triggers tremors, sweating, and nervousness and can send your heart racing at high speeds.

When do all these symptoms strike? The brains of most breakfast skippers start to short out around nine or ten o'clock in the morning. That's when low blood sugar levels give you a serious case of brain drain, causing your powers of reasoning and intelligence to take a nosedive. When your body reacts with an adrenaline kick, you'll probably begin to sweat and tremble. Hopefully, you won't be making an important presentation, taking a test, or doing anything really meaningful when you start feeling nervous and intellectually inept, because it could really mess up your day, your career, or maybe even your life. Your mother was right: breakfast really is the most important meal of the day.

Kids Need Their Morning Meal

While adults need to eat breakfast each day to perform their best, kids need it even more. Their growing bodies and developing brains rely heavily on the regular intake of food. When kids skip breakfast, they can end up going for as long as eighteen hours without food, and this period of semistarvation can create a lot of physical, intellectual, and behavioral problems for them.

Breakfast Is Brain Food

Scientists can explain the precise physiology of breaking the fast, but teachers can tell you firsthand about the impact of skipping breakfast on late-morning behavior and school performance. Breakfast is brain food: it's the meal most directly linked to academic achievement. Kids who skip breakfast have been found to have shorter attention spans, do worse in tasks requiring concentration, and even score lower on standardized achievement tests than kids who eat a morning meal.

A recent Harvard study lends support to the notion that hungry kids have more behavioral, attendance, and academic problems than children who are properly nourished. When they studied the effects of a breakfast pilot program in six Minnesota schools, they discovered that the kids participating in the breakfast program experienced a significant boost in learning and achievement. The breakfast eaters demonstrated a general increase in math grades and reading scores and showed significant improvements in their attention spans and conduct. In addition, kids who routinely ate breakfast enjoyed better health, making fewer visits to their school nurses than children who regularly missed the morning meal.

A Good Investment

If you and your kids regularly skip breakfast in the interest of saving time or getting a few more minutes of sleep, remember that eating a wholesome, nutritious morning meal will probably save you time in the long run. By recharging your brain and your body, you'll be more efficient in just about everything you do. Interestingly, studies show that kids who skip breakfast are tardy and absent from school more often than children who eat breakfast on a regular basis. Preparing a good breakfast can be as quick and easy as splashing some milk over cereal. Time invested in breakfast is much more valuable than the few extra minutes of sleep you might get by bypassing the morning meal. If you and your kids seem unable to make time for breakfast, consider enrolling your children in a school breakfast program, if possible, or pack a breakfast brown-bag the night before so that you and your kids can eat on the way to school and work.

Break the Fast to Shed the Pounds

Some people skip breakfast in an effort to lose weight, but the practice is more likely to cause weight gain than weight loss. Skipping breakfast is strongly linked to the development of obesity. Studies show that overweight and obese children, adolescents, and adults are less likely to break the fast each morning than their thinner counterparts.

According to research, skipping meals, especially breakfast, can actually make weight control more difficult. Breakfast skippers tend to eat more food than usual at the next meal or nibble on high-calorie snacks to stave off hunger. Several studies suggest that people tend to accumulate more body fat when they eat fewer, larger meals than when they eat the same number of calories in smaller, more frequent meals. To teens, especially teenage girls, skipping breakfast may seem like a perfectly logical way to cut down on calories and lose weight. It's important for moms to educate their kids about the importance of the morning meal and the role it plays in maintaining good health and preventing obesity.

The Emotional Benefits

While eating breakfast is undoubtedly good for your physical health, several studies have shown its importance in emotional health. People who regularly partake of the morning meal are more likely to have a greater degree of satisfaction in life, be less depressed and anxious, and experience lower levels of perceived stress than folks who regularly skip breakfast.

Start Them Off Right

Knowing the importance of breakfast doesn't make it any easier to convince kids with groggy morning appetites to eat it. Some kids seem to have stomachs that wake up a lot later than they do. Breakfast will go down more easily if you make eating last on the list of things to do in the morning rather than asking kids to eat when they first climb out of bed. For kids who just can't face food first thing in the morning, try sending them off to school with a brown bag full of dry breakfast cereal, a small carton of milk, and a piece of fruit.

Be Flexible

Although some kids bypass breakfast because they don't feel hungry in the morning, others decline simply because they don't like the traditional breakfast foods. Since breakfast is *when* you eat and not *what* you eat, you may have more success getting kids to eat if you offer them nontraditional breakfast foods. A bowl of soup or pasta or a hearty sandwich may seem a lot more appealing than the same old selection of cereals, Pop-Tarts, or breakfast bars.

Choose Wisely

Although you and your kids can eat a variety of nontraditional breakfast foods at the morning meal, the nutrients that those foods provide are important. Foods that are rich in complex carbohydrates are much better for your health—and your weight-loss efforts—than foods that are loaded with fat.

A recent study published in the *International Journal of Food Science and Nutrition* compared the effects of two breakfast meals containing an equal number of calories. One was rich in carbohydrates, while the other was high in fat. Volunteers eating the high-fat breakfast reported getting hungrier earlier in the day, which led them to start snacking before lunch. As a result, their total daily caloric intakes went up during the study. In contrast, subjects eating the high-carbohydrate breakfast were able to wait longer before eating again. As a bonus benefit, they performed better on tests requiring memory and concentration, and they reported feeling more alert and energetic throughout the day.

A similar study compared the effects of two calorically similar breakfasts. The total caloric content of the two meals was roughly equal, but one contained about 6 grams of fat, while the other offered about 28 grams of fat. Volunteers consuming the high-fat breakfast were found to have higher blood levels of glucose and insulin after eating, factors that can lead to obesity, as well as an increased risk of heart disease and stroke.

Eating breakfast has also been shown to decrease the risk of catching colds and other upper respiratory tract infections and improve health status in general.

Make Breakfast a Family Affair

The early-morning meal provides a window of opportunity for parents to nurture their children's development, both physically and emotionally. In bygone days, the evening meal provided the opportunity for families to gather around the table to share not only food but also the news and events of their daily lives. With work, after school activities, and sports practice often overflowing into the evening hours, many families now find it nearly impossible to eat dinner together. These days, it is estimated that fewer than 15 percent of American families eat their evening meals together on a regular basis.

One way that working moms can preserve the important tradition of breaking bread together is to make breakfast the meal that draws the family close. While your children may be scattered far and wide during the evening hours, it's a pretty safe bet that they're all in one place first thing in the morning. Making breakfast the main family meal may take a little adjustment at first, especially for the night owls in your family, but the extra effort is well worth it. In addition to providing much-needed family time, setting the alarm thirty minutes earlier each morning will ensure that everyone has time to eat at a more leisurely pace. The morning routine will likely become a little less frantic, eliminating some of the typical arguments as siblings vie for bathroom time and parents urge their kids to hurry, hurry, hurry. Kids will have more time to dress and gather up the things they'll need for school and after-school activities. Moms will have a few extra minutes to prepare wholesome lunches for family members or put a meal in the Crock-Pot for dinner. Most importantly, parents and kids can start the day as a family, reestablishing their unity and providing love, support, and encouragement to one another.

Optimize Your Morning Nutrition

Set mealtimes, especially for breakfast, make kids and adults less likely to snack throughout the day. They also help ensure that everyone gets the necessary nutrients for a well-balanced diet. Eating almost anything for breakfast is better than eating nothing, but as long as you're taking the time to eat, you might as well try to optimize your morning nutrition. A well-balanced breakfast should include one item from at least three of the five food groups. Since you'll want to eat a meal that is rich in complex carbohydrates, breakfast is an excellent time to eat whole-grain foods, which will also help you meet your daily fiber needs. If you and your kids eat a serving or two of fruit and vegetables each morning, meeting your requirements for five servings a day will be a lot easier. Breakfast is also an excellent time to take in some calcium-rich dairy products, like milk, yogurt, and cheese.

Calcium

Breakfast is a great time to work at least one glass of calcium-rich milk into the daily diet, whether it's drunk from a glass or poured over cereal. Kids need plenty of calcium while they're young to build strong bones and teeth. During childhood and adolescence, kids' bodies readily absorb calcium from the foods that they eat and pack it into their growing bones. In their youth, children's bodies are storing calcium in their bones, building calcium savings accounts for the future. It's important for them to get enough of the mineral in their daily diets so that their savings accounts will be large enough to serve as a retirement fund in their advancing years, protecting them from osteoporosis and bone fractures.

If you're an adult, you may not drink as much milk as you did while still a kid, but getting enough calcium is just as important as it ever was. Men and women need calcium at every stage of life. Around the midthirties, adults' bones reach their maximum size and strength, a state known as the peak bone mass. At this point, the body stops building bone and simply tries to hold on to what it has got. In folks who don't take in enough dietary calcium as middle-aged adults, bone mass begins to dwindle.

Men and women lose bone mass most rapidly in the fifth decade of life, but the process is accelerated in menopausal women when estrogen levels wane. Low-calcium diets speed bone loss even more. If enough bone is lost, osteoporosis develops, and bones become brittle and break easily.

Most people realize the importance of calcium when it comes to preventing osteoporosis, but calcium has other important health benefits. People who eat calcium-rich diets are less likely to develop high blood pressure than those with calcium-poor diets. Recent research bears good news for women who suffer from premenstrual syndrome. In a landmark study involving over 450 women diagnosed with premenstrual syndrome, supplemental calcium alleviated symptoms like bloating, food cravings, and pain by nearly half. In the last decade, scientists have also discovered that a high-calcium diet can cut your chances of getting colon cancer and reduce your risk of developing type II diabetes.

Getting enough calcium in your diet is especially important when you're trying to lose weight. Scientists at the University of Tennessee's Department of Nutrition recently happened upon this earthshaking discovery while they were studying the effects of dietary calcium on high blood pressure. When overweight and obese patients with high blood pressure followed a high-calcium diet, their blood pressure readings dropped significantly. But curiously, so did their weight. The patients lost an average of eleven pounds of body fat in one year.

The researchers surmised that the extra calcium must have been responsible for the unexpected weight loss. To test their theory that high-calcium diets promote weight loss, they designed a new study. This time, their subjects were overweight mice.

Some of the mice in the study were treated to the equivalent of the typical American fare, with low levels of calcium. Other mice consumed diets that contained moderate or high levels of calcium. Although the mice dined on the same number of calories, those with the greatest calcium intake lost the most weight—up to 33 percent of their total body weight.

Even better, the high-calcium diets seemed to rev up their metabolic rates. This energized metabolic state allowed the mice to burn fat, even while they were resting. In the mice consuming the high-calcium diets, fat breakdown was three to five times greater than that of the mice eating the low-calcium diet.

Additional studies have proven that calcium is capable of recharging the human metabolism as well. A recent trial demonstrated that patients following low-calorie diets lost more weight when they ate a healthy variety of low-fat dairy products. In a sixteen-week period, the folks on the low-calorie, high-calcium diets lost about fifteen pounds, while their low-calorie-, low-calcium–consuming counterparts lost less than four pounds.

In an analysis of over seven thousand men and women involved in the most recent National Health and Nutrition Examination Survey (NHANES III), researchers found that the men and women with the highest intakes of dietary calcium had the lowest body weights, even when calorie consumption was equal.

All this evidence leaves little doubt that dietary calcium plays a key role in preventing obesity and promoting weight loss. But there's a catch—calcium is most beneficial when it's obtained from the foods in your diet, not from supplemental pills, powders, or potions.

For an unknown reason, calcium from real food has a much greater positive impact on health and weight loss than calcium supplements. This phenomenon has been observed in numerous studies. Dietary calcium is better than supplemental calcium when it comes to preventing colon cancer, high blood pressure, type II diabetes, and osteoporosis.

In spite of all the perks that calcium offers, most folks don't get nearly enough in their diets. Children of ages four to eight years need 800 milligrams of calcium a day, and kids between the ages of nine and eighteen need at least 1300 milligrams daily. Unfortunately, most children and adolescents take in less than 800 milligrams of the mineral daily. The typical American adult consumes only about 600 milligrams a day, while most need more along the lines of 1,000 mg. If you're a nursing mother, a menopausal woman, or just getting on in years, it's a good idea to aim for an intake of 1,500 mg a day.

If you and your kids aren't getting as much of the mineral as you need, don't have a cow. It's never too late to start boning up on calcium intake, and milk and dairy products are excellent sources. Even low-fat milk and dairy products are calcium-rich, with a single serving offering roughly 300 milligrams. The food industry is helping boost calcium intake in Americans by fortifying orange juice, bread, and breakfast cereals with the mineral.

The bad news for adults is that even if you manage to meet or exceed your daily requirement for calcium, your body may not be able to use it. While the growing bodies and bones of kids and adolescents are equipped to absorb dietary calcium with ease, calcium isn't as readily absorbed from the adult bowel. Your body has to work a little harder at it, and it won't even try unless you give it a reason. Weight-bearing exercise, like light weight lifting or walking, is all the stimulus most adults need to trigger calcium absorption.

Lactose Intolerance—Be Wary of the Dairy

Milk has been called nature's "perfect food." But while it may be perfect for babies and small children, many older kids and adults can't stomach it. An estimated 50 million people in the United States have lactose intolerance, a condition that renders them unable to digest the sugars in milk.

The primary sugar in milk is lactose, a large, bulky molecule made up of two simpler sugars. Before lactose can be absorbed through the walls of the intestines and converted into energy for the body, it must be split into its smaller constituents. Splitting the sugar lactose is a relatively simple process, but it requires a special enzyme called lactase. In most folks, the enzyme is produced in adequate amounts by the lining of the intestine.

Almost all healthy infants make plenty of the enzyme, but as they're weaned from milk or formula, their lactase production naturally begins to slack off. In people with lactose intolerance, production of the enzyme can cease altogether.

Lactase production is a genetically programmed process, and whether or not you have lactose intolerance depends to a large degree on your heritage. As many as 70 percent of African-Americans, 90 percent of Asian-Americans, and 95 percent of Native Americans can't properly digest dairy products because they don't make enough of the enzyme lactase.

For the most part, the enzyme deficiency is permanent and irreversible, and if you're lactose intolerant, you'll stay that way for the rest of your life—unless, of course, you're a woman and you happen to get pregnant. Some 44 percent of lactose-intolerant women will temporarily regain the ability to digest the milk sugar during their pregnancies.

If your body doesn't produce enough lactase to digest the dairy products you consume, most of the milk sugar will remain undigested in the small intestine. And there it sits, acting like a sponge and drawing fluid into the bowel. The undigested sugar in a quart of milk can absorb up to a quart of water from outside the intestine, and voilà, you'll have intestinal cramping and diarrhea. The symptoms can start within fifteen minutes of drinking milk or eating dairy foods, although they may take several hours to develop.

The gastrointestinal discomfort may not be the worst of it, at least as far as your social life is concerned. The normal bacterial residents of your intestines devour the undigested lactose sugar, shamelessly forming gas as a by-product. The excess gas in your belly can lead to bloating and give you a killer case of cramps. And when the gas makes its inevitable exit, it can make you very unpopular with the people around you.

Surprisingly, many people with lactose intolerance aren't even aware that they have the problem—they don't associate their intestinal fireworks with the consumption of milk products. How do you know if you're lactose intolerant? Your doctor has several high-tech, high-priced tests available to help you find out. The least expensive way to make the diagnosis is simply to adopt a lactose-free diet for a few weeks. If most of your cramping, bloating, gas, and diarrhea disappears, you've probably got lactose intolerance.

If you find that you don't have the intestinal fortitude for milk, you don't have to give up dairy products altogether. Since lactose intolerance affects people in varying degrees, you may just need to experiment a little to find out exactly how much lactose you can tolerate before your gastrointestinal tract rebels. You'll probably be able to squeeze in a glass of milk or two a day, especially if you drink it with your meals. Consuming dairy products in modest amounts and with other foods, like breakfast cereals, helps hold the milk sugar in your stomach longer, increasing the chances that it will be digested. Most people with lactose intolerance can enjoy aged cheeses like Swiss and extra-sharp cheddar, as these foods contain only traces of lactose. And because yogurt contains helpful bacteria that have already begun the process of lactose digestion, you'll probably be able to eat it without any problems.

Thanks to modern technology, lactose-reduced dairy products are available in most supermarkets and health food stores. You can also find commercially prepared lactase supplements, such as Lactaid and Dairy Ease.

These supplements work just like your own natural enzyme, breaking down milk sugar into its smaller constituents so that you can eat dairy foods without suffering.

Lactose intolerance is a condition that you can live with. With a little extra effort, you can enjoy nature's "perfect" food without being perfectly miserable.

Breakfast Cereals

The new "Nutrition Facts" labels on packaging have made it a lot easier for moms to choose the most nutritious breakfast cereals for themselves and their children. A quick glance at the label gives you a good idea of how much saturated fat, cholesterol, dietary fiber, and sugar a breakfast cereal has to offer. No matter how good the nutrition labels look to conscientious moms, kids are likely to ignore them completely. They're more interested in the cartoon characters on the packages and the promise of the free toys inside.

Aware of this phenomenon, cunning cereal manufacturers strike below the belt, bypassing moms and aiming directly for their gullible kids. Kids are bombarded with television advertisements for sugary breakfast cereals that are virtually fiber free, artificially flavored and colored, and loaded with preservatives and additives. It's up to moms to deliver the message that what the cereal contains in terms of nutrients is actually more important than the dazzling packages and the free toys on the inside.

It's okay to allow your kids to pick a cool new cereal every now and then, even if it's not a nutritional superstar. You can allow them to eat it on occasion, like on weekend mornings or another prearranged day of the week. Even the "worst" cereals are made better with a serving of low-fat milk, and they're still far superior nutritionally to many other traditional high-fat breakfast foods, like doughnuts and sweet rolls.

On most days of the week, it's a good idea to stick with cereals that provide a little sound nutrition, or try to talk your kids into a mixture of two cereals. By mixing a high-sugar cereal like Frosted Flakes with one that's more nutritious, like Bran Flakes, you know they're at least getting a little fiber and reducing their sugar consumption. Since the cereals' ingredients

(continued on page 116)

Report Card for Breakfast Cereals*

A+

Very low sugar, low-fat, high-fiber cereals. One serving provides 1 teaspoon (5 grams) or less of sugar, 3 grams or less of fat, and 5 grams or more of fiber.

General Mills Fiber One

Kellogg's All-Bran Extra Fiber

Kellogg's All-Bran Original

Nabisco Shredded Wheat
(Regular or Spoon-size)

A

Cereals with very low sugar, low fat, some fiber. A single serving offers 1 teaspoon or less of sugar, 3 grams or less of fat, and 0 to 4 grams of fiber.

General Mills Cheerios

General Mills Kix

General Mills Total Corn Flakes

General Mills Total Whole Grain

General Mills Wheaties

Kellogg's Corn Flakes

Kellogg's Crispix

Kellogg's Product 19

Kellogg's Rice Krispies

Kellogg's Special K

Ralston Corn Chex

Ralston Rice Chex

B

Cereals that are high in fiber, low in fat. One serving has 5 grams or more of fiber, 3 grams or less of fat, and 1 to 4 teaspoons of sugar.

Kellogg's Bran Buds

Kellogg's Complete
Oat Bran Flakes

Kellogg's Frosted Mini-Wheats

Nabisco Frosted Wheat Bites
and 100% Bran

Post Fruit & Fibre Dates, Raisins,
Walnuts

Post Grape-Nuts

Post Premium Bran Flakes

Raisin Brans

Ralston Multi-Bran Chex

C and D

Cereals with more than 3 grams of fat.

General Mills Cinnamon
    Toast Crunch
General Mills Raisin Nut Bran
Kellogg's Blueberry Morning
Kellogg's Cracklin' Oat Bran

Kellogg's Great Grains Raisin,
    Date, Pecan
Post Banana Nut Crunch
Quaker 100% Natural Oats,
    Honey, & Raisins

F

Low in fiber, high in fat and sugar. One serving offers less than a gram of fiber and 2 teaspoons or more of sugar.

General Mills Cocoa Puffs
General Mills Reese's Puffs
General Mills Trix
Kellogg's Cocoa Rice Krispies
Kellogg's Frosted Flakes
Kellogg's Pop-Tarts

Post Cocoa Pebbles
Post Fruity Pebbles
Post Honey-Comb
Post Waffle Crisp
Ralston Cookie-Crisp
    Chocolate Chips

*Adapted from material compiled by *Consumer Reports*.

are listed in descending order by amount, you can get a general idea about what's really inside. Start with the sugar content. Some breakfast cereals, especially those made for children, contain 35 to 50 percent sugar. In terms of sugar content, eating these types of cereals is the equivalent of having a couple of chocolate chip cookies or a slice of cake for breakfast.

If the cereal offers more than 6 to 9 grams of sugar per serving, you should probably reject it as a breakfast staple. The American Dietetic Association is even stricter, recommending that you choose cereals with no more than 6 grams of sugar per serving. Cereals containing morsels of real dried fruit are the exception to the rule. Dried fruit boosts the cereals' sugar content, but they make up for it with added nutritional benefits, like extra vitamins and fiber.

Don't be lured into buying a sugary, low-fiber cereal just because it's packed with the entire alphabet of vitamins. As a consolation prize to nutrition-savvy mothers, most cereal manufacturers supplement their products with extra nutrients. Even so, an impressive lineup of vitamins and minerals doesn't make up for some cereals' high sugar and artificial ingredient content—not to mention the fact that the only way you'll get fiber from the product is if you eat the boxes they're packaged in.

To make sure that your kids are getting the most from the morning meal, look for words like "whole-grain" before ingredients like rice, corn, or barley on the box. This means that they're probably a reasonable source of complex carbohydrates. The Food and Drug Administration recently approved the following health claim for whole-grain foods, including breakfast cereals: "Diets rich in whole grain foods and other plant foods and low in total fat, saturated fat, and cholesterol and may reduce the risk of heart disease and certain cancers." To be able to make this claim, a cereal must contain at least 51 percent whole grain by weight, and list some type of whole grain as its first ingredient. The food must also be low in fat, with no more than 3 grams of fat per serving.

Most cereals, even the nutritionally deplete, sugary ones, are naturally low in fat, with granola cereals and those containing coconuts being the exceptions. These cereals can contain as much as 8 grams of fat in a single 1-ounce serving. They may not be as bad as they look on first glance, as they typically provide lots of fiber. The fat contained in many of these cereals is often unsaturated fat, which isn't as detrimental as fat of the saturated variety.

When it comes to counting the calories and other nutrients provided by breakfast cereals, be sure to consider the amount you actually consume, rather than the recommended serving size. Most people pile their cereal bowls with at least twice the amount recommended. If you're eating more than the suggested serving size, be sure to multiply the calories and other nutrients by the appropriate amount. Studies show that most folks prefer presweetened cereal. If you choose an unsweetened variety and then load it with sugar, don't forget to add 15 calories for each teaspoon of sugar that you pile on.

The Report Card for Breakfast Cereals on page 114 is based on the *Consumer Reports* comparison of more than one hundred top-selling cereals. Because cereal ingredients change from time to time, be sure to check the nutrition labels before you buy.

Eggs

While breakfast cereals are an excellent source of carbohydrates, and some provide a decent amount of fiber, most of them are low in protein. If you're looking for a breakfast food that's wholesome and rich in protein, don't forget about eggs.

Many moms try to steer their kids away from eggs, and it's no wonder. For the past fifty years, the American Heart Association has been encouraging people to cut down on their egg consumption. Eggs are cholesterol-rich, and eating them was once believed to elevate cholesterol levels dramatically.

Being the law-abiding, health-conscious citizens that we are, we've tried to comply with the recommended egg-restricting rations, and the egg has become somewhat of a forbidden food. But as it turns out, eggs really aren't all that bad for you. The latest research confirms what many experts have suspected for a while. If you and your kids are reasonably healthy, eating an egg a day won't necessarily drive up your cholesterol levels or your risk of heart disease.

Studies show that the cholesterol contained in foods doesn't have as great an effect on blood cholesterol as was once believed. The most important factors determining whether you have high cholesterol levels are the genes you inherited from your parents as well as the amount of saturated fat in your diet.

That's not to say that eggs aren't cholesterol rich. A large egg contains roughly 213 milligrams of cholesterol, an amount that provides about two-thirds of the recommended daily allowance. All foods obtained from animal products have some cholesterol—the fat-like substance is found in every human and animal cell. Your body produces all the cholesterol it needs, and if you eat too many high-cholesterol foods, you might end up with high cholesterol levels in your blood, which can clog your arteries and increase your risk for heart disease and stroke.

Even if you've been diagnosed with high cholesterol levels, it's reasonable to include up to four eggs a week in your diet. If you've never had a problem with your cholesterol levels, eating an egg or two won't corrode your arteries or cause you to fall over dead from a heart attack. If you're healthy, your body can compensate for a little extra cholesterol in your diet by slacking off on its own production. If your cholesterol level is higher than either you or your doctor would like, you still don't have to swear off eggs altogether. You just have to approach the yolk of the egg with a little extra caution, since it contains the entire 213 milligrams of cholesterol, and 6 grams of fat, to boot. The egg white, on the other hand, is still your dietary friend. Two egg whites have just 35 calories, and they're totally devoid of fat and cholesterol.

Although the egg has long been vilified, it's actually a rather admirable food, containing a veritable smorgasbord of important nutrients. Each egg offers around 6 grams of protein, providing roughly 12 percent of the U.S. Department of Agriculture's Recommended Daily Value for that nutrient. Egg protein is of such high quality that it is often used as the gold standard by which other types of protein are measured.

A single egg contains varying amounts of thirteen vitamins, plus several important minerals. The yolk of the egg is one of the few food sources of vitamin D, an ingredient that helps your body absorb calcium to build strong bones and teeth. A large egg packs only about 75 calories. If you're still worried about the cholesterol content, you can console yourself with the fact that many of the egg's heart-healthy nutrients, like folic acid and antioxidants, have important benefits that offset the negative effects of cholesterol on your heart.

If you seem unable to overcome your deeply ingrained egg phobia, you can always turn to egg substitutes, a route that more and more Americans are taking these days. Egg substitutes first hit the market in 1973, and today they account for roughly a quarter of America's egg consumption. Egg substitutes are a low-fat, low-cholesterol alternative to the real thing, with no messy shells for moms to clean up.

Juices

Although you don't want your kids drinking too many high-calorie drinks throughout the day, breakfast is an excellent time to offer them 100 percent fruit juice. Drinking juice with the morning meal helps you and your children get a jump on the day's fruit intake, and sometimes, drinking juice in the morning is a little easier to manage than eating the fruit itself. When you're shopping for fruit juices, be sure to look for the words "100% fruit juice" on the label. Words like "beverage," "ade," or "drink" are a good indication that the product is mostly sugar water flavored with a splash of real fruit juice.

Vitamin C

Most citrus fruit juices are rich sources of vitamin C. A single serving typically provides 100 percent of the day's requirements for the nutrient: 90 milligrams for men and 75 for women.

Vitamin C is an important nutrient for several reasons. It facilitates the absorption of iron from other foods and plays a key role in the production of red blood cells. These actions make it useful in the prevention and treatment of iron-deficiency anemia.

Vitamin C is essential for the proper functioning of the body's immune system. The nutrient increases production of white blood cells, enabling your body to fight off colds and other infections. It also enhances respiratory function by disarming histamine, a substance that can trigger allergy and asthma attacks.

Studies show that the higher the level of vitamin C in your bloodstream, the lower your risk of heart disease. The vitamin improves the ability of your arteries to dilate in times of stress, promoting proper blood flow to your heart. By reducing cholesterol deposits along artery walls, it also helps prevent atherosclerosis, or hardening of the arteries.

Diabetics can benefit from taking vitamin C, since it seems to help regulate insulin release and slow diabetes-related damage to eyes, nerves, and kidneys. Vitamin C has been shown to reduce the formation of gallstones, protect smokers from toxins in cigarette smoke, and improve mental function in elderly adults.

Vitamin C's greatest claim to fame is its ability to serve as a powerful antioxidant. Antioxidants are thought to cleanse the body of free radicals, high-energy oxygen molecules that disrupt cells and damage tissues. These renegade molecules contribute to degenerative conditions, such as arthritis, cancer, cataracts, and heart disease.

With all its attributes, it's easy to think that if some vitamin C is good for you, more is better. But if you and your kids are eating the recommended five servings of fruits and vegetables a day, you're already getting all the vitamin C your body can use, and supplements aren't really necessary. Since vitamin C is water-soluble, it can't be stored in the body's fat deposits, and any excess is simply excreted in the urine. For this reason, it is essential for you and your kids to meet your body's requirements for vitamin C each and every day.

Folic Acid

In addition to being rich in vitamin C, many fruit juices are excellent sources of folic acid. Folic acid is the man-made version of folate, a B vitamin found naturally in dark green vegetables, citrus fruits, and some animal products. Folic acid in the diet is converted to folate in the body.

A growing body of evidence suggests that the B vitamin may help prevent heart disease. Folic acid has the unique ability to clear the blood of a harmful chemical called homocysteine, which has been shown to contribute to hardening of the arteries. Recently, homocysteine has been added to the growing list of risk factors for heart disease—just as important and detrimental as high cholesterol levels, high blood pressure, cigarette smoking, or obesity.

The results of several studies suggest that an adequate intake of folic acid can cut the risk of heart disease by half. Drinking a single serving of citrus fruit juice will allow you and your children to get an entire day's supply. If you have a bowl of cereal or a piece of toast with your juice, that's even better. Since 1998, manufacturers of prepared foods like breakfast cereals and breads have been fortifying their products with folic acid. The good news is that your body absorbs the synthetic folic acid found in fortified foods nearly twice as well as it absorbs the natural folates contained in your diet.

The Recommended Daily Allowance (RDA) for folate is 400 micrograms of synthetic folic acid, in addition to the folate that occurs naturally in your diet. Women of childbearing age should consume more, along the lines of 800 micrograms a day, to prevent birth defects of the brain and spinal cord in their unborn children.

Almost all fruit juices are wholesome additions to a well-balanced breakfast, but a few standouts are worth mentioning. Purple grape juice is one of the nutritional superstars. Not only is it loaded with vitamins, the tasty treat has been shown to help reduce the risk of heart disease. Components in purple grape juice appear to reduce the stickiness of platelets in the blood, an effect that can help prevent the formation of blood clots in the arteries leading to the heart.

Drinking purple grape juice may also help lower the risk of many types of cancer. According to the U.S. Department of Agriculture, the juice has more than three times the antioxidants contained in other commonly consumed juices, and twice the antioxidant power of many fresh fruits and vegetables.

Some of the most potent antioxidants in purple grape juice are substances known as flavonoids. These agents have been shown to prevent the oxidation of low-density lipoprotein (LDL), the bad type of cholesterol, in the bloodstream. Oxidation of LDL creates plaques on the walls of arteries leading to the heart, restricting blood flow and contributing to the development of heart disease. If you're interested in improving the heart health of yourself and your kids, purple grape juice is an excellent choice.

Cranberry Juice

If you or any of your children are plagued by urinary tract infections, you'll definitely want to squeeze a glass of cranberry juice into your morning meal. Drinking cranberry juice is a proven, doctor-approved home remedy for warding off infections of the kidneys and bladder. Although it was once believed that drinking cranberry juice helped kill invading bacteria by acidifying the urine, scientists have recently found that substances called condensed tannins in the juice are responsible for its medicinal properties.

These agents are capable of preventing infection-causing bacteria from attaching to cells in the kidneys and bladder by stunting the growth of hairlike filaments on their surfaces. Without these Velcro-like appendages, the bacteria aren't able to attach themselves to the cells lining the urinary tract, and they're more likely to be flushed out of the body with urination.

This anti-adhesion property of cranberry juice is also being explored for its role in dental and digestive health. Early research suggests that the compounds in cranberries prevent the bacteria responsible for periodontal gum disease from sticking to teeth. Preliminary data also show that cranberries may have a similar effect on *H. pylori*, the bacterial source of some stomach ulcers.

Cranberries are also being praised for their protective properties against heart disease. Like grape juice, cranberry juice is loaded with antioxidant flavonoids that interfere with the oxidation of cholesterol.

The oil from the cranberry seed is rich in heart-healthy omega-3 fatty acids and a specific type of vitamin E. Both agents have been shown to lower cholesterol and triglyceride levels, as well as reduce the clotting potential of the blood. The antioxidant action of the vitamin E in cranberries is also being exploited for its cancer-fighting effects. In mice injected with human cancer cells, daily consumption of cranberry juice has been shown to thwart the development of tumors.

While the role of cranberry juice in preventing heart disease and cancer is still under investigation, there's no doubt that it is extremely effective in warding off bladder and kidney infections. As a preventive measure, experts recommend drinking at least three ounces of cranberry juice cocktail on a daily basis. Cranberry juice isn't a cure for urinary tract infections, but when it comes to preventing the condition, a few ounces of cranberry juice may be worth a pound of antibiotics.

Grapefruit Juice

While almost all types of fruit juice are nutritious additions to any breakfast, kids and adults who take medicine on a regular basis should approach grapefruit juice with a little caution.

There's no doubt that grapefruit juice can be part of a healthy diet. Like orange juice, the tart and tasty beverage has no fat, cholesterol, or refined sugar, and it's packed with vitamins and minerals. A single serving provides 100 percent of the recommended daily allowance for vitamin C, and it's an excellent source of folate.

The juice carries the American Heart Association's official stamp of approval—it contains compounds that may reduce the risk for cardiovascular disease and cancer. The juice has been found to lower blood levels of low-density lipoprotein (LDL) cholesterol, a substance known to contribute to heart disease.

But there's a downside to guzzling grapefruit juice. In a study at the Harvard School of Public Health, researchers found that a daily eight-ounce serving of grapefruit juice was associated with a 44 percent increase in the risk of kidney stone development. Of the seventeen beverages assessed, grapefruit juice was associated with the highest increase in risk, surpassing tea, colas, and other citrus juices.

If you take certain medications, grapefruit juice may be hazardous to your health in another way. Nearly a decade ago, researchers investigating drug interactions made an interesting discovery. Grapefruit juice appeared to have a significant impact on how the body absorbs and degrades certain medicines.

Drinking just one cup of grapefruit juice can lead to a whopping ninefold increase in the concentration of certain drugs in the bloodstream. Among the drugs found to react to grapefruit juice are some medicines used to treat hypertension, certain hormones, antihistamines, sedatives, and several drugs used to treat high cholesterol. As research continues, additional drugs are being added to the list.

Not only does grapefruit juice increase the concentration of certain drugs in the bloodstream, it also delays their elimination from the body. Both actions can increase the frequency and intensity of medication side effects. Scientists have pinpointed the agent responsible for the problem. Naringin, the component that gives the grapefruit its characteristic bitter taste, also appears to interfere with the absorption and elimination of some medications. Naringin blocks the action of enzymes in the liver and small intestine that are responsible for drug degradation. Other citrus fruits don't contain naringin—the substance is unique to whole grapefruits and grapefruit juice.

For most folks, grapefruit juice is a wholesome addition to a healthy diet. But for some, it can be a bit of a health hazard. If you or your kids have kidney stones or take medications, ask your doctor before making grapefruit juice a regular part of your morning meal.

Action Plan

✔ **Make breakfast a family affair.** Ask your kids if they'll be willing to try getting together for breakfast on a regular basis. Explain the reasons that breakfast is important to their health and school performance and tell them that you'd like to spend more time together as a family. Ask for their help in specific ways, like agreeing to get up thirty minutes earlier than usual and meeting at the kitchen table at a set time in the morning. If your plan isn't met with unanimous approval, you can compromise by designating a few mornings of the week as Family Breakfast Days, leaving them to their own devices on the remaining mornings. When kids see how much better they feel and how organized and pleasant mornings can be, they'll be more likely to want to eat breakfast with the family on a regular basis.

✔ **Plan ahead.** Ask your kids what they'd like to eat for breakfast. Take a few minutes the night before to set the table and gather ingredients and supplies that you'll need for the morning meal. Also, ask your kids to get their clothes and school supplies ready the night before so they'll be able to enjoy breakfast with the family at a leisurely pace.

✔ **Set a good example.** Make sure that you sit down and eat with your family to show them that you believe that the nutrition provided by breakfast is important not only to kids but to adults as well.

✔ **Leave clean-up for later.** Since spending time together as a family is more important than having a spotless kitchen, consider just rinsing off breakfast plates and dishes and leaving them in the sink. You can assign kids kitchen duty on a rotating basis as an afternoon chore or allow them to earn extra money by washing dishes and cleaning the kitchen after school.

✔ **Make breakfast a positive event.** Use your time together to coordinate family schedules, encourage kids in their school efforts, and praise them for their accomplishments. If your children will be coming home from school to an empty house, encourage them to exercise and finish their homework rather than watch TV or spend the afternoon on the computer. If schedules permit, plan an evening meal or a fun fitness activity for the family.

Breakfast Cone

1	plain ice cream cone
¼	cup fat-free yogurt
¼	cup sliced fruit
2	tablespoons crunchy cereal

Add fruit to yogurt; mix. Pour mixture into ice cream cone; top with cereal.

Servings: 1 **Calories per serving:** 124

G-Factors per serving: Fat 0, Carbohydrate 14, Protein 17

Applesauce Oatmeal

1	package instant oatmeal, any flavor
½	cup applesauce

Prepare oatmeal as directed; add applesauce.

Servings: 1 **Calories per serving:** 164

G-Factors per serving: Fat 4.5, Carbohydrate 14, Protein 17

Mexican Omelet

2	large egg whites
½	cup frozen vegetables
¼	cup grated low-fat cheese
2	tablespoons salsa
	Nonstick vegetable spray

Heat vegetables in microwave until warm. Lightly coat skillet with vegetable spray; cook egg whites. Top eggs with salsa; place vegetables on top; sprinkle with cheese. Fold in half.

Servings: 1 **Calories per serving:** 137

G-Factors per serving: Fat 5, Carbohydrate 8, Protein 15

PB&B Breakfast Sandwich

2   slices fat-free whole-wheat bread

1   tablespoon reduced-fat peanut butter

½   banana, thinly sliced

Toast bread; smooth on peanut butter; top with sliced bananas.

Servings: 1   **Calories per serving:** 107

G-Factors per serving: Fat 6.5, Carbohydrate 7, Protein 4

Green Eggs and Ham Sandwich

2   egg whites

6   slices (1 serving) lean deli ham

2   drops green food coloring

2   slices fat-free whole-wheat bread

    Nonstick vegetable spray

Add food coloring to eggs. Lightly coat skillet with vegetable spray; scramble. Serve with ham on toasted bread.

Servings: 1   **Calories per serving:** 214

G-Factors per serving: Fat 1.5, Carbohydrate 26, Protein 24

String Cheese Breakfast Sandwich

1   stick string cheese

6   slices (1 serving) low-fat deli meat

1   slice fat-free whole-wheat bread

Roll meat slices around cheese; wrap with bread.

Servings: 1   **Calories per serving:** 174

G-Factors per serving: Fat 5.5, Carbohydrate 14, Protein 17

Cantaloupe Fruit Bowl

½   small cantaloupe

½   cup fat-free yogurt

½   cup pineapple chunks in juice

Spoon yogurt into cantaloupe half; top with pineapple.

Servings: 1   **Calories per serving:** 236

G-Factors per serving: Fat 0, Carbohydrate 43, Protein 16

Breakfast Bagel

1   whole-wheat bagel

2   tablespoons fat-free cream cheese

2   tablespoons 100% fruit preserves

Toast bagel; top with cream cheese and fruit.

Servings: 1   **Calories per serving:** 153

G-Factors per serving: Fat 1, Carbohydrate 30, Protein 6

Fabulous French Toast

2   slices fat-free whole-wheat bread

1   egg white

2   tablespoons skim milk

¼   teaspoon cinnamon

1   tablespoon powdered sugar

     Nonstick vegetable spray

Blend egg white, milk, and cinnamon in mixing bowl. Lightly coat skillet with nonstick spray; place on stove on medium heat. Dip bread slices in egg mixture; remove excess; place on skillet to brown. Turn bread and brown on opposite side. Sprinkle with powdered sugar.

Servings: 1   **Calories per serving:** 152

G-Factors per serving: Fat 0, Carbohydrate 28, Protein 10

Fruity Oatmeal

1   package instant oatmeal, fruit flavor

½   cup sliced bananas or fresh or frozen berries

Prepare oatmeal as directed. Top with fruit.

Servings: 1   **Calories per serving:** 195

G-Factors per serving: Fat 2.5, Carbohydrate 40, Protein 3

Fruit Smoothie

1   cup fat-free plain or vanilla yogurt

¼   cup 100% fruit juice

½   cup fresh strawberries

Pour ingredients in blender; blend until smooth. Let kids experiment with different flavors of yogurt, 100% fruit juice, and fresh or frozen fruits.

Servings: 1   **Calories per serving:** 172

G-Factors per serving: Fat 0, Carbohydrate 33, Protein 10

Breakfast Pita

2   egg whites

1   tablespoon salsa

¼   cup frozen vegetables

¼   cup lean ham or turkey cubes

¼   cup grated low-fat cheese

1   whole-wheat pita, cut in halves

Cook egg whites in microwave; set aside. Heat frozen vegetables, meat chunks, cheese, and salsa in microwave. Add mixture to eggs; place in pita halves.

Servings: 2   **Calories per serving:** 188

G-Factors per serving: Fat 4.5, Carbohydrate 17, Protein 20

Applesauce Waffles

1	fat-free frozen waffle
½	cup applesauce
¼	teaspoon cinnamon

Toast waffle; top with applesauce. Sprinkle with cinnamon.

Servings: 1   **Calories per serving:** 116

G-Factors per serving: Fat 0, Carbohydrate 26, Protein 3

Peanut Butter Banana Wrap

1	slice fat-free whole-wheat bread
½	banana
1	tablespoon reduced-fat peanut butter

Spread peanut butter on bread; wrap around banana half.

Servings: 1   **Calories per serving:** 224

G-Factors per serving: Fat 5.5, Carbohydrate 35, Protein 8.5

Breakfast Taco

1	4-ounce baked boneless, skinless chicken breast, shredded
2	egg whites
¼	cup reduced-fat Mexican cheese mix, grated
2	tablespoons salsa
¼	cup each chopped tomato, lettuce, pepper
2	warmed taco shells

Scramble egg whites; place egg whites and shredded chicken in warmed taco shell. Top with cheese, salsa, and veggie mix.

Servings: 2   **Calories per serving:** 228

G-Factors per serving: Fat 8.5, Carbohydrate 11, Protein 27

Fruit Pita

1   whole-wheat pita, cut in half

½   cup fat-free cottage cheese

½   cup pineapple chunks

Toast the pita halves. Stuff with cottage cheese and fruit.

Servings: 2   **Calories per serving:** 140

G-Factors per serving: Fat 0, Carbohydrate 26, Protein 9

Peanut Butter and Banana Smoothie

½   cup fat-free vanilla yogurt

1   tablespoon reduced fat peanut butter

½   banana

1   plain ice cream cone

Slice banana and place in blender. Add peanut butter and yogurt; blend until smooth and creamy. Serve in ice cream cone.

Servings: 1   **Calories per serving:** 223

G-Factors per serving: Fat 5.5, Carbohydrate 35, Protein 8.5

Strawberry Waffle Stacks

3   round fat-free frozen toaster waffles

4   tablespoons fat-free strawberry-flavored soft cream cheese

1½   tablespoons strawberry preserves

1   medium banana, sliced

1   cup sliced strawberries

Toast waffles according to package directions. Place 1 waffle on plate; spread with 2 tablespoons cream cheese and half of the preserves. Arrange one half of the banana and half of the strawberries on top. Top with another waffle; repeat layer with remaining ingredients; place remaining waffle on top. Cut waffle stack into quarters. Garnish each quarter with sliced strawberries.

Servings: 2   **Calories per serving:** 228

G-Factors per serving: Fat 0, Carbohydrate 48, Protein 9

Blueberry Bran Muffins

1⅓   cups bran cereal

¾   cup fat-free milk

¼   cup egg substitute

2   teaspoons vanilla

1   cup flour

⅓   cup firmly packed light brown sugar

1   tablespoon baking powder

1   tablespoon baking soda

¾   teaspoon cinnamon

¾   cup fresh or frozen blueberries

In a medium-size mixing bowl, combine bran cereal, milk, egg substitute, and vanilla. Let stand 5 to 10 minutes. In a large bowl, combine flour, brown sugar, baking powder, baking soda, and cinnamon. Add cereal mixture to flour mixture and mix well. Stir in blueberries; spoon mixture into paper-lined muffin tins and bake for 30 minutes at 325 degrees F until muffins are slightly browned.

Servings: 8 muffins; 1 muffin = 1 serving   **Calories per serving:** 161

G-Factors per serving: Fat 1, Carbohydrate 30, Protein 4

Chapter 7

Fast but Good

The super-sizing of Americans can be blamed, in large part, on our growing love affair with fast food. Nearly half of every food dollar spent by American families goes to restaurants. Each year in the United States, hungry patrons shell out over $110 billion for the fattening fare, spending more money on burgers and fries than on personal computers and new cars. The average American admits to eating at least three meals a week in fast food restaurants, an unhealthy indulgence that contributes not only to obesity but to dozens of other medical maladies as well.

A Nutritional Black Hole

While fast food is tasty, convenient, and relatively inexpensive, it has some serious shortfalls in the way of nutrition. Even taking into account the lettuce and tomato on your favorite burger and the potatoes in french fries, fast food meals fall far short of providing the recommended allotment of fruits and vegetables necessary for good health.

The U.S. Department of Agriculture recommends eating at least five or more servings of a variety of fruits and vegetables each day. People whose diets are rich in fruits and veggies have lower rates of heart disease and most types of cancer than those whose diets are lacking fresh foods. Sadly, American children now get about one quarter of their total vegetable servings in the form of french fries or potato chips.

The recommended intake of fiber is around 30 grams each day, yet a typical fast food meal offers only around 5 grams, putting Americans at risk for developing heart disease and diabetes, as well as some serious gastrointestinal problems, including constipation, diverticulosis, and even colon cancer. Unless you and your kids make a habit of eating the cardboard containers that hold your fries, diets that are rich in fast food are probably poor in fiber.

While fast food has some serious nutrition omissions in the way of beneficial nutrients and fiber, it is typically loaded in calories, and the caloric content has risen steadily over time. In the 1940s, when the first fast food restaurant made its debut, a typical meal including a burger, fries, and a soft drink offered about 450 calories. The same meal today—in super-sized proportions—provides around 1,500 calories. For some folks, this number fulfills or surpasses their entire daily caloric need. Eating this many calories in one sitting promotes weight gain for another reason. The human body is capable of processing only about 800 calories at any one meal before the excess calories are stored as fat.

The "More Is Better" Fallacy

At the urging of fast food manufacturers, kids are quickly learning that more is better. Burger King and McDonald's recently began offering bigger versions of their kids' meals, appropriately named the "Big Kids Meal" and the "Mighty Meal," respectively. For less than a dollar extra, kids can purchase double hamburgers and cheeseburgers instead of singles, or an order of six fried "nuggets" containing reconstituted chicken parts and pieces instead of the usual four. Marketers for the food chains say they're really just trying to be helpful, offering kids aged eight to ten years old the ego boost and the extra food their growing bodies' "need." Thanks to this type of entrepreneurial altruism, American kids will be primed to sing out "super-size it!" by the ripe old age of twelve. With younger and younger kids developing the gastric capacity and intestinal fortitude to conquer the weightiest of the super-sized meals, they're sure to face a fast food letdown in adolescence or early adulthood. Undoubtedly, the fast food industry is already hard at work developing the next generation of giant meals, so that our children will be able to say "mega-size it!" or "industrial-size it!" by the time they're in their twenties.

Although most kids have learned to relish the salty, greasy gustatory delights of burgers and fries, the food itself usually isn't the biggest attraction of fast food restaurants. Many kids want the Happy Meal primarily for the much-advertised, highly glamorized plastic toy that comes packaged with it.

It may surprise you to know that fast food joints are among the world's largest distributors of toys. McDonald's alone distributes more than 1.5 billion toys a year, beating out full-time toy companies like Hasbro and Mattel. The promise of these pint-size pieces of plastic lures more than 90 percent of American kids between the ages of three and nine to McDonald's restaurants every month.

Even minus the toy, a Happy Meal with a burger, fries, and small soda still serves up 640 calories. Although rich in calories, the meals are seriously lacking in the nutritional stuff most important for growing kids, including fiber, calcium, and fruits and vegetables. Worse yet, they're loaded with fat and cholesterol. Research has demonstrated that kids and adults who regularly partake of fast food consume significantly greater amounts of fat than folks who tend to dine at home. With 40 percent of its calories supplied by fat, fast food can contribute to high cholesterol levels, hardening of the arteries, and heart disease.

Even if you're a careful, gram-counting consumer, you may still be getting more fat, cholesterol, and calories than you bargain for. That's because the nutritional information provided to you by the well-meaning purveyors of fast food may not always be completely accurate. While your favorite super-deluxe cheeseburger may call for a level teaspoon of mayonnaise, the frenzied folks preparing your meal don't always have time to make leisurely measurements. After all, you want your fast food fast, right? So it shouldn't come as any surprise to you that the folks behind the grill don't take the time to measure out precisely two perfectly level tablespoons of special sauce and spread it neatly on your burger. These highly trained food service technicians often use the culinary equivalents of squirt bottles, paint brushes, and caulking guns to dispense high-fat condiments like butter and mayonnaise to your food. As a result, the actual amounts of the greasy garnishes that end up on your sandwich may differ significantly from the amounts that are recommended by the top chefs back at the restaurants' headquarters. One slip of the culinary caulking gun, and you could end up consuming double the amount of fat, cholesterol, and calories that you intended.

For moms who are determined to pass up the drive-through window, it's helpful to carry a well-stocked cooler or picnic basket in your car whenever you and your kids are on the road. When children clamor to be fed, you can whip out individual servings of nutritious finger foods like cut- up fruits and vegetables, yogurt, or sandwiches. This will save you a little extra time and expense and save your kids a lot of unnecessary fat and calories.

Ordering Tips

If you find that the very survival of you and your kids seems to depend on the occasional consumption of fast food, you don't have to cut it out altogether; you just have to make judicious, nutritious choices.

Order Food to Go. You can reduce the associated fat and calorie content by a significant degree eating the food at home rather than at the restaurant or atop the dashboard dining facilities in your car. Studies show that people tend to consume more food when they're eating away from their own kitchen tables. When you bring fast foods home, you can supplement the meal with side orders of fresh fruits and vegetables, saving yourself 15 to 30 grams of fat by simply foregoing the fries. Instead of guzzling the 32-ounce soda that comes with the meal, you can opt for a glass of water, saving yourself around 300 calories and several tablespoons of sugar.

Avoid Buffets. If you want to keep your fast food and your good health, avoid all-you-can-eat buffets like the scourges to humanity that they are. If this type of establishment holds any appeal for you at all, you might be able to diminish it a significant degree by just spending a few minutes in the parking lot, watching the portly patrons come and go. Chances are that you won't see too many thin, healthy-looking folks frequenting these modern-day shrines to gluttony.

Forego the Fries. When you're eating out, you'll have some important decisions to make. A super-sized serving of french fries may have as many as 30 grams of fat. For some folks, this is almost an entire day's supply. Are the fries worth it? If they are, then you might decide to just go for it. But if they aren't, you'll need to forget the fries and stick with the leaner choices on the menu.

Stick to the "Light" Menu. Most fast food restaurants offer "light" menus and low-fat selections. You're always better off choosing from among these items. Fried foods and those served with high-fat condiments like mayonnaise, "special" sauce, and tartar sauce need to be approached with extreme caution. If the restaurant doesn't offer a light menu, your best bet is to choose salads with low-fat dressings or grilled chicken sandwiches. When it comes to ordering soups, choose the broth-based varieties rather than those that are cream-based.

Don't Be Afraid to Special-Order. Wherever you end up eating, ask for all condiments to be served on the side rather than slathered on your food by the chef, who is likely to be as indifferent to the lining of your arteries as he is to the circumference of your waistline. A single tablespoon of regular mayonnaise or salad dressing contains about 9 grams of fat and 100 calories, so you'll want to use these condiments sparingly, if at all.

Although vegetables are usually safe choices, their nutritional value is significantly diminished if they're overcooked to the point of disintegration or if they're swimming in lakes of oil or butter. Ask for your vegetables to be served plain and lightly steamed, so that they'll be reasonably nutritious and free of added fat.

If you're in the mood for pasta, ask if you can have your pasta served plain with the sauce on the side, so that you can apply it to your noodles a little more sparingly than the chef might see fit.

Fear the Fryer. While fish and chicken entrees sound nutritionally safe, you have to pay attention to the methods in which they are prepared. The fried versions of either food put them in the same class as burgers, and drowning fish or chicken in creamy sauces or butter can demote them to the nutritional status of high-fat desserts. To ensure that they remain low in fat and cholesterol, order your fish or chicken entrees baked or grilled.

Take Charge of Your Plate. Even when you're dining at restaurants that don't offer super-size versions of their normal fare, you can bet that a "single" serving still provides enough calories for at least two meals. The average restaurant meal contains around 1,500 calories, even minus the bread and dessert. It's a good rule of thumb to leave at least a third of the meal on your plate—some for Mr. Manners and the rest for Mrs. Health. Or, you can eat half of your meal while you're at the restaurant and save the other half for the next day's lunch.

It's always a good idea to opt for smaller portions than the ones provided, and you can be fairly certain that you won't run the risk of starving. Some restaurants are happy to oblige your request for half-orders. If they aren't, you can try ordering a child's plate of the same meal. If that doesn't work, you and your dinner date can always share an entree. If you feel that you must indulge in a food that is high in fat and calories, don't make matters worse by committing the twin sins of eating the wrong kind of food *and* eating too much of it. As you lose weight and gain health, you'll be pleased to find that savoring just a few bites of a tasty treat is often every bit as satisfying as stuffing yourself with a half-pound serving. It's definitely less guilt-provoking.

Beware the Salt Overload

One of the worst things about eating out is that you have little to no control over the salt content of your food, and the foods offered by most restaurants are typically loaded with the stuff. If your doctor has recommended that you or your kids lower your sodium intake, you'll definitely want to limit your consumption of fast foods. A burger and an order of fries can contain well over 2,000 milligrams of sodium, allowing you to meet almost your entire daily allowance in one sitting. Even the most innocent-looking condiments aren't safe: pickles and ketchup are loaded with salt.

Most of us realize that excess dietary salt can endanger our health, but try as we might, we're still having trouble shaking the salt habit. Despite the wide variety of newfangled low-sodium foods and revealing nutrition labels, Americans' salt consumption hasn't changed much over the last century.

Table salt is a chemical composed of two minerals: sodium and chloride. Most healthy folks require less than 500 milligrams of sodium a day, the amount in about a quarter teaspoon of salt. Unfortunately, it takes more than just a pinch to satisfy our salt cravings, and the average American consumes 3,000 to 6,000 milligrams of sodium a day, for a grand total of ten to fifteen pounds of salt each year.

All this salt can take a toll on your health, driving your blood pressure up to a dangerous degree. About a fourth of Americans currently have high blood pressure, a condition that increases the risk of strokes and heart attacks. Even small increases in blood pressure can dramatically raise the risk of death.

As it turns out, some people can effectively lower their blood pressure simply by cutting back on their salt consumption. Although the current recommended daily allowance for sodium is 2,400 milligrams a day, many experts now believe this number is too high.

In a study known as the DASH (Dietary Approaches to Stop Hypertension) trial, volunteers who followed the recommended diet and limited their sodium consumption achieved significant reductions in blood pressure. Subjects who consumed 1,500 milligrams of sodium a day lowered their systolic blood pressures (top numbers) by an average of 11.5 points, while their diastolic blood pressures (bottom numbers) fell by an average of 7.1 points. These reductions in blood pressure are comparable to those offered by many prescription medications.

Most physicians now agree that all Americans—even those with normal blood pressure—can benefit by cutting back on salt. Holding the salt could help prevent the rises in blood pressure that typically occur with weight gain in kids and adults.

If you're watching your salt intake, eating out can be risky business. Walking into the typical fast food restaurant is like entering a salt mine. You can cut your salt consumption by ordering foods with no added salt. If your taste buds rebel, you can spice things up with herbs and other low-

(continued on page 144)

Best Picks and Nixes for Fast Food Choices

Next time you have to swing by a drive-through, here's a little guide for what to look for and what to avoid.

	Carbohydrate grams	Protein grams	Fat grams
Arby's			
Go for:			
Light Roast Chicken Deluxe	33	24	7
Light Roast Turkey Deluxe	33	20	6
Light Roast Beef Deluxe	33	18	10
Avoid:			
Chicken Breast Filet	42	22	23
Regular Roast Beef	35	22	18
Curly Fries (small)	40	4	16
Burger King			
Go for:			
BK Chicken Whopper (no mayo)	29	20	10
Hamburger	28	14	10
Cheeseburger	28	16	14
Avoid:			
Chick'N Crisp Sandwich	37	16	27
Whopper Jr.	28	19	24
Whopper	46	27	31
Whopper with Cheese	46	33	39
Double Whopper	47	49	59
Double Whopper with Cheese	47	55	67
Bacon Cheeseburger	27	24	22
Onion Rings	38	5	19
French Fries	43	5	20
Ocean Catch Filet	33	16	28
Bacon, Egg & Cheese Croissanwich	20	19	22

	Carbohydrate grams	Protein grams	Fat grams
Dairy Queen			
Go for:			
Single Hamburger	29	17	13
French Fries (small)	31	4	13
Avoid:			
Hot Dog	23	9	16
Hardee's			
Go for:			
Hamburger	33	10	10
Cheeseburger	34	12	14
Chicken Filet	50	19	13
Avoid:			
Quarter Pounder Cheeseburger	34	29	29
Fisherman's Filet	50	23	21
Kentucky Fried Chicken			
Go for:			
Tender Roast Sandwich (no sauce)	23	31	5
Corn on the Cob	35	5	2
Mashed Potatoes (½ cup)	12	3	2
Avoid:			
Chunky Chicken Pot Pie	69	29	42
Popcorn Chicken (large)	36	30	40
Honey BBQ Pieces (6)	33	33	38
McDonald's			
Go for:			
Hamburger	35	13	9
Cheeseburger	35	16	13
Chicken McGrill (no mayo)	45	26	7

(continued on page 144)

Best Picks and Nixes for Fast Food—continued

	Carbohydrate grams	Protein grams	Fat grams
McDonald's—continued			
Lean Deluxe	35	22	10
French Fries (small)	26	3	10
Egg McMuffin	28	18	11
Scrambled Eggs	1	12	10
Hash Browns	15	1	7
Hot Cakes	44	3	2
Avoid:			
Big Mac	45	26	32
Big Xtra	51	24	46
Big Xtra with Cheese	52	29	55
Crispy Chicken	54	23	50
Chicken McGrill	46	26	18
Filet-O-Fish	45	15	26
Quarter Pounder	37	23	21
Quarter Pounder with Cheese	38	28	30
Taco Bell			
Go for:			
Bean Burrito	54	13	11
Tostada	27	10	12
Hard Taco	11	10	11
Beef Soft Taco	18	12	12
Grilled Chicken Soft Taco	20	4	7
Grilled Steak Soft Taco	19	14	7
Grilled Steak Soft Taco Supreme	21	15	11
Soft Taco Supreme	22	11	13
Big Beef MexiMelt	22	15	15
Steak Gordita Supreme	27	17	14
Chicken Gordita Supreme	28	16	13
Double Decker Taco	37	14	15

	Carbohydrate grams	Protein grams	Fat grams
Chili Cheese Burrito	40	13	13
Avoid:			
Nachos	34	5	18
Mexican Pizza	43	28	48
Steak Gordita Baja	27	17	18

Wendy's

Go for:

Grilled Chicken Sandwich	35	27	8
Jr. Cheeseburger	34	17	13
Spicy Chicken Sandwich	43	28	15
Avoid:			
Bacon Cheeseburger	26	30	24
Fish Sandwich	42	18	25
Chicken Nuggets (6)	12	14	20
Big Bacon Classic	46	34	30
Chicken Club Sandwich	44	31	20
Breaded Chicken Sandwich	44	28	18
Single with Everything	37	25	20
Jr. Cheeseburger Deluxe	36	18	17
Jr. Bacon Cheeseburger	34	20	19

Pizza Hut

Go For:

Veggie Lover's Pizza (2 slices)	29	18	16
*Avoid:**			
Cheese Pizza (2 slices)	38	26	20
Pepperoni Pizza (2 slices)	40	24	22
Supreme (2 slices)	40	30	28

*In general, avoid the folowing pizza varieties: Pan Pizza, Stuffed Crust, The Big New Yorker, and the Chicago Dish.

sodium seasonings. It may take a while to adjust to the taste of a low-sodium diet, but with a little patience and persistence, you can shake the salt habit for good.

When you're eating out, it's helpful to go armed with a little knowledge about the nutrient values of some of the items on the menu. If you're eating a balanced diet that provides around 2,000 calories a day, your G-Factor for fat will be 44. In order to distribute your fat grams equally among your meals and snacks, you'll probably want to limit your fat intake at each meal to about 15 grams.

Action Plan

- ✔ **Eat in more often.** You're less likely to overeat when you eat at home, so make eating at home a priority. If you prepare home-cooked meals that are hassle-free, you'll be less tempted to eat out.

- ✔ **Resist the temptation to super-size it.** More food for less money isn't really such a great deal, especially if you and your kids don't need the extra calories.

- ✔ **Choose grilled chicken sandwiches and hold the mayo.** Grilled chicken offers a lot less fat and fewer calories than beef or deep-fried fish. Simply leaving off the mayonnaise can save you 9 grams of fat and 100 calories per teaspoon.

- ✔ **Forego the fries.** French fries are loaded with fat, salt, and calories, and they are virtually free of any beneficial nutrients. Instead of ordering fries, opt for a plain baked potato or a side salad with fat-free dressing.

- ✔ **Prepare for dashboard dining.** When you're on the go and meal-time rolls around, having a cooler packed with nutritious snacks in the car will allow you to eat on the run without resorting to fast food. If you must stop for food, try swinging by the grocery store instead of a fast food restaurant. You can dash in and pick up some tasty finger foods, like fresh fruit, squeeze yogurt, lean deli meat, and whole-wheat crackers or bagels.

Chapter 8

Smart Snacks

Snacking has gotten a bad rap. Mention the word "snack," and visions of sugary cookies, greasy chips, and fizzy sodas begin to dance through most mothers' heads. But in spite of its negative connotations, snacking the *right* way is actually a good thing. Snacks can make a big contribution to the daily nutrition of kids and adults of all ages.

Adults may think they have to eat three squares a day and avoid between-meal snacking in order to lose weight. But snacks happen, so you might as well spend some time planning and preparing for them. Seventy-five percent of adults eat at least one snack a day, while 91 percent of children engage in snacking on a regular basis.

Snacking Done Right

The real problem with snacking isn't *when* you snack or even *if* you snack—it's what type of foods you choose to eat. When approached properly, snacking contributes to weight loss rather than weight gain. Eating small amounts of nutritious foods between meals is an excellent way to stave off hunger and prevent overeating at mealtime. If you eat a whole apple in the midafternoon hours, you'll probably be less likely to overeat at your evening meal. The 100 calories and the satisfaction that you get from the apple may end up saving you 500 or so extra calories that you might be tempted to devour at dinnertime, when you're extremely hungry.

Smart snacking also promotes weight loss by revving up your metabolism, the rate at which your body burns calories. When you supply your body with food on a regular basis, the wheels of your metabolic machinery keep turning at a steady clip. With calories continuing to come in predictably, your body never finds it necessary to slip into an energy-saving, crisis mode.

If you think of your metabolism as a calorie-consuming fire, it makes a little more sense. To keep a fire burning, you have to add fuel, like wood, on a regular basis. If you wait too long to add wood to the fire, it will go out. If you dump huge quantities of wood on the fire all at once, on the other hand, you'll smother the fire. The same is true with your metabolism. If you don't fuel your body with small amounts of nutritious foods regularly throughout the day, your body will begin to conserve energy by slowing your metabolic rate. Your metabolism will also slow if you go for long periods without eating and then dump a huge meal into your body. Eating small, frequent meals and snacks regularly throughout the day is the best way to keep your metabolism humming.

Most kids like to snack, and moms should encourage the practice by providing a variety of nutritious foods and plenty of opportunities to eat them. Snacking is a perfectly natural human behavior that begins at birth, when babies nurse frequently throughout the day. As kids get older, they still need to eat often. The high energy needs and growing bodies of toddlers and preschoolers make snacking between meals more of a necessity than a luxury. Their limited stomach capacity makes it nearly impossible for them to get all the calories and nutrients they need from just three meals a day. As kids enter school, they continue to have high energy needs relative to their small sizes. Eating as often as six times a day is not only normal, it's ideal. Providing your children three regular meals and two or three between-meal snacks is an excellent way to make sure they're getting the nutrition they need for optimum growth and development.

The catch is that snacks should *contribute* to the total nutrient intake of the day, rather than *detract* from it. Kids get approximately 25 percent of their daily calories from snacks, so it's important to make sure that the foods they eat are wholesome and nutritious. Snacks should fill in nutritional gaps and make up for foods and nutrients that were missed at breakfast, lunch, and dinner. If your child manages to finish most of her meat and vegetables at lunch, but loses interest before she gets around to eating her fruit or drinking her milk, it's not a big deal. You can always make up for the missed nutrients at the next snack simply by offering her foods like fresh strawberries and yogurt or sliced apples and cheese. Snack time also provides an excellent opportunity to offer new foods to kids in a fun, low-pressure situation.

While the practice of snacking is a good one, most of the foods that we commonly consider snack foods are not. Left to their own devices, many kids make poor choices at snack time, choosing high-fat sweets and fried, salty foods over more nutritious fare like fresh fruit and vegetables, yogurt, and sandwiches.

In an effort to prevent weight gain in themselves and their children, moms may be tempted to purchase reduced-calorie snack foods that are sugar-free or low in fat. Interestingly enough, in the same time frame that Americans have seen an explosion of fat-free, reduced-fat, and sugar-free snack foods on supermarket shelves, obesity in children and adults is at an all-time high.

While few scientific studies have addressed this paradox, a likely explanation for this trend is that kids and adults may tend to overcompensate when they eat foods that are low in fat or calories. It's only natural to rationalize that as long as you're eating low-fat or sugar-free foods, you should be able to eat as much as you like. Another possible explanation is that you may not experience the same degree of satiety from foods that are lacking in most nutrients. While eating two or three "real" chocolate chip cookies may fill you up, it may take an entire box of reduced-fat or sugar-free chocolate chip cookies to satisfy your hunger.

Research has shown that artificial sweeteners in low-calorie foods may actually stimulate your appetite rather than satisfy it, due to a phenomenon known as the cephalic phase response. Studies have found that when humans eat foods that taste sweet, the brain signals the pancreas to secrete insulin in preparation for the storage of calories that will undoubtedly follow. Because there are few—if any—calories in some artificially sweet-ened foods and beverages, the insulin is left roaming around your blood with no energy to store and nothing to do. It is thought that the presence of extra insulin in your bloodstream actually sends a feedback signal to the brain, which, in turn, stimulates your appetite.

Some artificially sweetened foods can be a valuable part of a well-bal-anced diet for older kids and adults. Sugar-free yogurt is a good example. While the sweet taste of artificially sweetened yogurt may trigger the cephalic phase response and the release of insulin from the pancreas, it's not a big deal. Once the insulin is loose in your bloodstream, it will find plenty of work to do because even sugar-free yogurt provides plenty of calories and nutrients. On the other hand, artificially sweetened sodas aren't all that beneficial. When the sweet taste of diet cola triggers the cephalic phase response, the insulin that is released from your pancreas won't find any nutrients to store because diet colas are totally devoid of car-bohydrates, protein, and fat. As a result, the energy-seeking insulin remains at large in your bloodstream, stimulating your appetite and leading you to eat or drink again, whether you need to or not.

It's not a good idea to eat dessert foods at snack time on a regular basis, but occasionally, your sweet tooth might absolutely demand a treat. To avoid getting caught in the aftermath of the cephalic phase response, your best bet is to just go ahead and eat a "real" nutrient-containing food rather than one that is artificially sweetened. This will allow you to snack, rather than graze, and there's a big difference between the two.

Grazing is unplanned, almost continuous eating that can last for hours, stretching from one meal to the next. Snacking, on the other hand, is a planned and scheduled event, with a clear beginning and a definite ending. The same rules that apply to meals apply to snacks. Snacks shouldn't be consumed in front of the television, and foods should be removed from their packages and served on or in the appropriate dish. Instead of grab-bing a whole king-size bag or box, you and your kids should serve your-selves appropriately sized portions and put the container back in the cupboard or fridge. Whenever possible, snacks should be eaten at the table in a leisurely manner.

Even when snacks are eaten on the run, moms can help make sure their kids get the nutrients they need by preparing ahead of time. It's a good idea to keep a well-stocked cooler or a picnic basket in your car. Kids may need to eat en route to ball practice, karate class, or other after-school activities. Having a variety of tasty, nutritious finger foods within arm's reach will make it a lot easier to drive by the drive-through window at your favorite fast food restaurant. It will also help keep extra fat and calories out of your kids' diets.

Whenever possible, snacks should be scheduled, even if loosely, so that kids know when to expect them. To ensure that kids are hungry when it's time to eat their regular meals, moms should try to provide snacks a couple of hours before the next meal and discourage snacking at other times throughout the day. Snacks should be planned as well-balanced mini-meals, emphasizing nutritious foods and beverages. The foods that you and your kids eat at snack time should add to the day's total intake of nutrients. To ensure that your snacks contribute to your health, rather than just pile on extra pounds, snacks should include one or two selections from the five food groups: fruits, vegetables, grains, meats and beans, or dairy. While you're striving to eat a well-balanced diet, you'll be eating more foods from the fruits and vegetables groups than any other food group, so it's a good idea to try to work them into snack time. This will make it a lot easier for you and your kids to get the recommended five servings a day.

As you might suspect, junk foods, which most Americans have come to equate with snack foods, do not belong to any of the five food groups. In spite of their deceptively wholesome name, Cheese Doodles don't really fall into the dairy group, any more than potato crisps or corn chips fall into the vegetable group. Cakes, cookies, and candy add little more than calories, sugar, and fat to the day's nutrient intake, so they aren't good caloric investments.

Liquid Snacks

Liquid intake has a profound impact on the overall nutritional status of American children, and obesity in kids has as much to do with what they drink as what they eat. Moms need to teach their children to make sensible beverage choices at snack time.

Soft Drinks

In the past few decades, soft drinks have become a national addiction. The average American adult now consumes about three hundred cans of the bubbly beverage each year, and grown-ups aren't the only ones who obey their thirst. In the last twenty years, teenagers have nearly tripled their soft drink consumption. In 1994, a U.S. Department of Agriculture survey revealed that the typical teenage boy consumed three 12-ounce cans of soda a day, while the typical teenage girl drank approximately two cans a day. Kids of ages six to eleven aren't far behind, drinking double what their counterparts did two decades ago. More than half of American eight-year-olds down at least one soft drink a day.

It's okay to have a Coke and a smile every now and then, but moderation is the key. In itself, a single serving of soda isn't all that bad for you; it just isn't all that good for you. A regular, unadulterated soft drink is loaded with sugar, caffeine, acids, and artificial dyes and flavors. But take away the calories, and its nutritional value is a big, fat goose egg.

The Sugar

Currently, soft drinks constitute the leading source of added sugar in the diet of children and adolescents. The U.S. Department of Agriculture suggests a maximum of 6 tablespoons of sugar a day for a child consuming 1,600 calories, the number necessary for most preschool children. With about 3 tablespoons of sugar per serving, a child gets almost half the daily recommended amount of sugar in just one drink. And while the average teen doesn't come close to meeting his needs for fruits, vegetables, or dairy products, he consumes about twice the recommended amount of sugar each day, mostly in the form of between-meal soft drinks.

It's not surprising that the trend of obesity in children and adolescents has risen steadily along with the increase in soft drink consumption. A child's chances of becoming obese increase by a factor of 1.6 for each additional daily serving of soda consumed. With around 160 calories in an average 12-ounce can of soda, just adding two cans a day to your normal diet can net you a weight gain of almost two and a half pounds a month. The link between sodas and obesity in children is so great that soft drink consumption can be used as a fairly reliable predictor of changes in Body Mass Index measurements.

Soft drinks promote obesity in children and adolescents more than any other type of food or beverage. Intrigued by this phenomenon, scientists have designed studies to determine the reasons behind it, and the results of their research offer a very plausible explanation. When human beings consume excess energy in the form of food at a given meal or snack, their bodies tend to compensate for the extra calories by reducing hunger at the next meal or snack. But this compensatory mechanism doesn't seem to be fully functional when excess calories are consumed in the form of liquids. If, for example, you begin taking in an extra 200 calories a day by eating a snack consisting of a sandwich or a cup of yogurt, you'll tend to reduce your caloric intake by the same amount at the next meal or over the course of the day. On the other hand, if you take in an extra 200 calories at snack time by drinking a soft drink, your body won't activate the same compensatory mechanisms, and you probably won't end up reducing your daily caloric intake at all. In the long run, you'll end up gaining weight.

In a study that helped prove the relationship between energy intake in the form of liquids and body weight, volunteers were given either a snack consisting of food or a single sugar-sweetened beverage each day for a period of three weeks. Their total energy intake and their body weight increased when they drank the sugar-sweetened beverages, but remained the same when they ate food that provided an equal number of calories. Similar studies have shown that kids who regularly consume soft drinks take in about 200 calories more each day than their counterparts who do not consume sodas on a regular basis.

In addition to obesity, a number of other negative health consequences have been attributed to the consumption of sugar-sweetened drinks. While no real link has been established between sugar consumption and hyperactivity in children, there's plenty of evidence to support the fact that it contributes to loss of tooth enamel and dental cavities. The combination of sugar and acid in soft drinks begins to dissolve tooth enamel after just twenty minutes of exposure.

The Caffeine

As if the added sugar in soft drinks isn't bad enough, there's also the caffeine content to contend with. Caffeine is totally lacking in nutrient value, and it doesn't really add taste, texture, or color to soft drinks. Caffeine affects kids and adults in a similar manner. As a stimulant, it can interfere with sleep and may affect the behavior of people who are overly sensitive to it. Because it acts as a diuretic, caffeine promotes the elimination of body water, and caffeine-containing beverages are especially poor choices for replacing fluids in hot weather or during exercise.

Caffeine is a double-edged sword when it comes to bone health in children. Even a can or two of soda a day can be dangerous when consumed during the peak bone-building years of childhood and adolescence. Kids who meet their fluid needs with caffeine-containing beverages are less likely to consume all the calcium they need from milk to build strong bones and healthy teeth. While the average child needs around 1,300 milligrams of calcium a day, most American kids get 800 milligrams or less. Low calcium consumption combined with a high caffeine intake spells double trouble for kids' bones. The caffeine content of many soft drinks contributes to bone loss, which can lead to bone fractures and the eventual development of osteoporosis. Other ingredients found in soft drinks, including sugar, phosphorus, and sodium, seem to interfere with kids' calcium absorption as well, making the mineral more likely to end up in the toilet than inside their bones where it belongs. A recent Harvard study found a strong link between cola consumption and broken bones in adolescents. Girls who drank colas on a regular basis were found to be five times more likely to suffer fractures than girls who chose caffeine-free beverages.

Further complicating caffeine consumption is the risk of addiction. Caffeine is one of the most widely consumed drugs in the world. For people who are dependent on the substance, missing a regularly scheduled dose can lead to a well-defined withdrawal syndrome, which includes headaches, irritability, and unhealthy rises in blood pressure. The fact that kids display signs and symptoms of caffeine withdrawal is a good indication that it may not be beneficial for their developing brains. If you want to give your children soft drinks at snack time every now and then, it's a good idea to choose those that are caffeine free.

It's not always easy to determine a product's caffeine content because manufacturers are not required to divulge this information on their nutritional labels. If a beverage contains caffeine, the manufacturer must list the substance on the label, but not necessarily the amount. Most colas contain anywhere from 35 to 38 milligrams of caffeine per 12-ounce serving. Diet colas often pack a more powerful punch than regular sodas. A 12-ounce can of Diet Coke has about 42 milligrams of caffeine, while the same amount of Coke Classic contains only 35 milligrams. A 12-ounce can of Pepsi One offers about 56 milligrams of caffeine, 18 milligrams more than the same amount of regular Pepsi or Diet Pepsi.

Soft drink manufacturers claim that small amounts of caffeine are added only for taste, not for the drug's power to keep addicts coming back for more. They say that the bitter taste of caffeine has the unique ability to enhance other flavors in their products. But many experts beg to differ. Blind taste tests conducted at Johns Hopkins Medical Institution found that only 8 percent of regular soft drink consumers could distinguish between regular and caffeine-free soft drinks.

Don't Forget About Water

Though not nutritious in the true sense of the word, water is an ideal liquid to give your kids at snack time. It has no calories, but it is still the most important substance your kids will put into their bodies. Water is vital to life, second only in importance to oxygen. Most healthy people can survive for weeks without food, but only three or four days without water. Water makes up a large percentage of the brain and the body itself. Since it is the primary ingredient of human beings, it's easy to see why drinking it is critical. A loss of just 5 percent of body water results in weakness and irritability and impairs concentration. A loss of just 15 to 20 percent can be fatal.

You and your kids need to drink plenty of water on a regular basis to stay healthy and fight disease. The mucous membranes that line the nose and throat are the first line of defense against invading viruses and bacteria. When these membranes are moist, they act like sticky flypaper, trapping and destroying germs before they can cause infection. Blood, which is roughly 85 percent water, delivers the cellular soldiers of the immune system throughout the body to help destroy disease-causing organisms. Water helps lubricate joints, cushion internal organs, and moisten eyes and skin. It carries food through the digestive tract, delivering nutrients and removing waste from cells and tissues.

If you don't adequately replace your fluids, your body will remind you by signaling you that you're thirsty. Oddly enough, the built-in sensation of thirst isn't a very reliable indicator of your body's state of hydration. You feel thirsty only after your body is considerably dehydrated and the salt content of your blood is increased. Salty blood pulls saliva from your mouth, making it feel parched and sending you in search of some liquid refreshment.

While the sensation of thirst comes only after you are partially dehydrated, it is often deactivated before you've satisfied your body's need for fluids. Just wetting your mouth can quench your thirst to a large degree, causing you to stop drinking long before you've met your body's fluid requirements. Because thirst isn't a reliable indicator of your body's state of hydration, you shouldn't count on it alone to regulate your fluid intake. Humans need about one quart of water a day for every fifty pounds of body weight, and soda, juice, and milk don't really count toward this requirement. Drinking water regularly throughout the day is the best way for you and your kids to stay ahead of your fluid requirements.

Smart Snacking Strategies

Kids begin choosing and preparing their own snacks fairly early in childhood, and this can be a mixed blessing for busy moms. Although it's an excellent idea to allow children to make their own selections at snack time, you'll spend a lot less time worrying about what they're eating if you've censored their selections ahead of time. When it comes to getting your kids to chose nutritious snacks, your best bet is to bring only those foods into your home that you feel good about them eating. If your kids can't find cookies, cakes, and chips in the kitchen, you won't find them snacking on these foods, at least while they're at home.

You can make it easier for children to choose and prepare their own nutritious snacks by making your kitchen a kid-friendly place. If you want to see how it's done by the pros, just take a stroll through your favorite grocery store. It will help if you crawl through the aisles on your knees, because this is where crafty grocers display kid-targeted foods. In your own kitchen, strategically placing nutritious foods front and center at eye level and within arm's reach of your kids will help you steer them in the right direction.

In the kitchen cupboard, you can fill the lower shelves with granola bars, whole-wheat bread and crackers, single-serving packages of oatmeal, microwave popcorn, and nutritious cereals. Keep a fruit bowl on the counter or tabletop and fill it with fresh apples, grapes, oranges, and bananas. Make sure your kids find lots of tasty treats in the cookie jar, like small packages of raisins, dried fruit, and trail mix.

In the fridge, stock plenty of yogurt, low-fat deli meat, string cheese, and fruit cups. Keep a variety of cut-up fruits and veggies within easy reach. If you package them in clear, single-serving plastic bags, they're more likely to get eaten. If you think your ravenous teen will take the extra time necessary to slice and dice the head of cauliflower you've stowed in the vegetable bin, you're probably dreaming. And while a big bunch of broccoli may not look even remotely edible to a child, a small package of bite-size broccoli florets and a squeeze bottle of fat-free dip may seem just about irresistible.

While you're in the fridge, throw out all the sodas and replace them with more wholesome beverages. Small boxes of 100 percent fruit and vegetable juice, bottled water, and low-fat milk are much better choices. In the freezer, make sure your kids find nutritious goodies like frozen yogurt, bagels, and prepackaged minimeals that are low in fat. Weight Watchers, Lean Cuisine, and other manufacturers offer a wide variety of low-calorie, nutritious frozen entrees. While these prepared foods take a back seat to home-cooked meals, they'll do in a pinch. From a nutrition standpoint, they're a lot better for you and your kids than frozen pizzas or burritos.

Making smart snacking the path of least resistance for your kids is one of the best ways you can ensure they're eating properly, even when you're not around to supervise.

Action Plan

✔ **Plan snacks, don't ban them.** Keep your kitchen stocked with nutritious foods that you won't mind your kids eating, and loosely schedule snacks about two hours before the next meal.

✔ **Give them a choice.** Allow your kids to choose between two or more similar foods. Don't set them up for failure by asking questions like, "Would you rather have a sweet potato or a bowl of ice cream for a snack?" Instead, offer them a choice between apple slices or orange sections, whole-wheat crackers or a bagel, celery sticks or baby carrots. This lets them exercise their powers of choice, but within your guidelines.

✔ **Choose age-appropriate snacks.** Kids younger than two should not be offered sugar-free, fat-free, or low-fat foods. Offer them nutritious snacks in appropriate sizes: about one tablespoon of a food for each year of age.

✔ **Check the labels.** When buying prepared snacks, be sure to check the labels. Low-fat foods may be very high in sugar, while those that are sugar free are often high in fat.

✔ **Offer plenty of variety.** If you serve up the same snacks over and over, your kids are likely to get bored and start making requests for foods like cookies and chips rather than the same old thing.

✔ **Vary the presentation.** Dress up fruits and vegetables for maximum kid-appeal. Cut food in fun shapes to make it harder to resist.

✔ **Allow your kids to be creative with their food.** Give them a few toothpicks so they can use fruit and vegetable chunks as building

blocks. Fill a squirt bottle with low-fat yogurt or salad dressing
and allow them to decorate their food. Fill a few saltshakers
with colored sugar sprinkles and allow them to add fun colors to
their snacks.

✔ **Try, try again.** If your child doesn't like a particular food the first
time around, try again later. It may take two, three, or even ten
tries before kids get used to new tastes and textures.

✔ **Set a good example.** Kids learn eating habits in the same way
they learn just about everything else: by imitating your behavior.
By choosing nutritious snacks for yourself, you're encouraging
your kids to do the same.

✔ **Let them participate.** Remember that kids like to eat what they
make, and they're more likely to try new foods if they helped
prepare them. Have them find new recipes to try out, looking in
cookbooks, magazines, or on the Internet. Once they find a food
they want to make, have them develop a shopping list. At the
supermarket, they'll have fun hunting for the necessary ingredients while they learn their way around the grocery store. Back
home, the fun of preparing the recipe is surpassed only by the
excitement of eating their creations.

Veggie Bowl

1	green, yellow, or red pepper
2	stalks celery, sliced and cut into 4-inch pieces
10	baby carrots
¼	cup fat-free salad dressing

Wash vegetables and slice celery. Cut top off pepper; remove seeds from inside to form veggie bowl. Pour salad dressing into veggie bowl and stack celery and carrots inside.

Servings: 1   **Calories per serving:** 132
G-Factors per serving: Fat 0, Carbohydrate 31, Protein 2

Instant Applesauce

2	small red apples
1	tablespoon lemon juice
1	teaspoon sugar
	dash cinnamon

Wash and peel apples, removing the core. Cut apples into small chunks. Place in blender with lemon juice; blend until smooth. Pour mixture into bowl; stir in cinnamon and sugar.

Servings: 1   **Calories per serving:** 136
G-Factors per serving: Fat 0, Carbohydrate 34, Protein 0

Pretzel Kabobs

½	ounce fat-free pretzel sticks
2	ounces baked lean ham or chicken chunks
1	ounce reduced-fat cheese, cut into chunks

Allow kids to build their own kabobs by skewering meat and cheese chunks with pretzels.

Servings: 1   **Calories per serving:** 275
G-Factors per serving: Fat 7, Carbohydrate 23, Protein 30

Fruit Kabobs with Dip

½ cup halved fresh strawberries

½ banana, sliced

½ cup grapes

½ cup pineapple chunks in juice

½ cup fat-free fruit yogurt

Let kids build their own kabobs by alternating fruit chunks on skewers. Dip in yogurt.

Servings: 1 **Calories per serving:** 236
G-Factors per serving: Fat 0, Carbohydrate 53, Protein 6

Mini Pizzas

½ whole wheat bagel

2 tablespoons spaghetti or pizza sauce

¼ cup grated low-fat cheese

¼ cup baked chicken chunks

Spread sauce on bagel; sprinkle with cheese; top with chicken chunks. Toast in oven or microwave until cheese melts.

Servings: 1 **Calories per serving:** 184
G-Factors per serving: Fat 4, Carbohydrate 21, Protein 16

Frozen Juice Pops

½ cup 100% fruit juice

½ cup pineapple chunks in juice

1 cup fat-free yogurt

Pour fruit, yogurt, and juice into blender; blend until smooth. Pour into 2 small plastic cups and insert a spoon; freeze.

Servings: 2 **Calories per serving:** 132
G-Factors per serving: Fat 0, Carbohydrate 29, Protein 4

Yogurt Parfait

1   cup fat-free yogurt, any flavor
1   cup sliced strawberries
½   cup crunchy cereal
¼   cup reduced calorie strawberry preserves

Allow kids to layer yogurt, fruit chunks, preserves, and cereal in tall dessert glasses. Eat now or refrigerate for later.

Servings: 2   **Calories per serving:** 180
G-Factors per serving: Fat 0, Carbohydrate 36, Protein 9

Trail Mix

½   cup granola or crunchy cereal
½   cup raisins
½   cup almonds, pecans, or walnuts
2   ounces chocolate chips
½   cup dried apples
4   ounces tiny fat-free pretzels

Mix and eat.

Servings: 6   **Calories per serving:** 267
G-Factors per serving: Fat 7, Carbohydrate 44, Protein 7

Veggie Platter

1   cup broccoli florets
1   cup cauliflower florets
1   cup baby carrots
1   medium green pepper, sliced
4   tablespoons fat-free dressing

Dip and eat.

Servings: 2   **Calories per serving:** 98
G-Factors per serving: Fat 0, Carbohydrate 20, Protein 4.5

Fruit Jell-O

1   package sugar-free, fruit-flavored gelatin
1   cup unsweetened sliced fresh or frozen strawberries
8   tablespoons reduced-fat whipped topping

Prepare gelatin as directed; add fruit. Pour into individual dessert cups and refrigerate until jelled. Top with whipped topping.

Servings: 4   **Calories per serving:** 64
G-Factors per serving: Fat 4, Carbohydrate 6, Protein 1

Fancy Animal Crackers

15 fat-free animal crackers
1   tablespoon reduced-fat peanut butter
1   teaspoon colored sugar sprinkles

Let kids spread peanut butter on their animal crackers and top with colored sprinkles.

Servings: 1   **Calories per serving:** 106
G-Factors per serving: Fat 2, Carbohydrate 21, Protein 2

Cookie-Cutter Sandwiches

2   slices fat-free whole-wheat bread
1   slice low-fat cheese
6   slices low-fat deli meat
1   leaf lettuce
1   thin slice tomato
    Cookie cutter

Let kids make their own special sandwiches by piling meat, cheese, lettuce, and tomato on bread. Help them cut their sandwiches into stars, gingerbread men, or hearts with cookie cutters—they're much more fun to eat!

Servings: 1   **Calories per serving:** 295
G-Factors per serving: Fat 6.5, Carbohydrate 33, Protein 26

Ants on a Log

2   stalks celery

1   tablespoon reduced-fat peanut butter

⅛   cup raisins

Wash celery stalks and cut into 4-inch pieces (logs). Spread peanut butter on stalks; place raisins (ants) in single file in peanut butter.

Servings: 1   **Calories per serving:** 169
G-Factors per serving: Fat 5.5, Carbohydrate 24, Protein 6

Tuna Salad Veggie Cups

1   pouch water-packed tuna (3 ounces)

2   tablespoons fat-free mayonnaise

2   tablespoons sweet relish

1   small green pepper

In small bowl, mix tuna, mayonnaise, and relish; set aside. Cut top from pepper; remove seeds to fashion a cup. Fill with tuna salad.

Servings: 1   **Calories per serving:** 192
G-Factors per serving: Fat 0, Carbohydrate 24, Protein 24

Apple Volcanoes

1   medium apple

1   tablespoon reduced-fat peanut butter

2   tablespoons raisins

2   tablespoons granola

Cut top off apple; remove core. Fill center with peanut butter; sprinkle with granola and raisins.

Servings: 2   **Calories per serving:** 247
G-Factors per serving: Fat 6.5, Carbohydrate 42, Protein 5

Italian Chicken Pitas

   1   4-ounce boneless, skinless chicken breast half, baked and cubed

  ½   cup reduced-fat chunky vegetable spaghetti sauce

   1   whole-wheat pita, halved and warmed

In bowl, stir together spaghetti sauce and chicken. Heat in microwave until warm; spoon into pita bread halves.

Servings: 2   **Calories per serving:** 216

G-Factors per serving: Fat 4, Carbohydrate 24, Protein 21

Butterfly Sandwiches

   1   4-ounce boneless, skinless chicken breast half, baked and shredded

   4   slices fat-free whole-wheat bread

   2   tablespoons fat-free ranch dressing

   2   4-inch carrot sticks

  ¼   cup raisins

In a small mixing bowl, mix chicken and ranch dressing; spread on bread to make sandwich. Cut sandwich into 2 triangles. Use a carrot stick for the body and raisins for the eyes.

Servings: 2   **Calories per serving:** 295

G-Factors per serving: Fat 2.5, Carbohydrate 44, Protein 24

Strawberry-Banana Smoothie

   1   large banana, peeled and sliced

   2   cups fresh or frozen unsweetened strawberries

   2   cups fat-free milk

   2   teaspoons vanilla

Place all ingredients in blender and process until smooth.

Servings: 4   **Calories per serving:** 109

G-Factors per serving: Fat 0.5, Carbohydrate 21, Protein 5

Chapter 9

What to Buy

Developing a smart food-shopping strategy is key to helping your kids stay healthy and lose weight. The food that you bring home from the grocery store determines what they will end up eating, and what you take with you on your trip to the grocery store often determines what you bring home. The only item that is more important than your checkbook is your shopping list; it's virtually impossible to avoid impulse buying without it. Before you head out to the supermarket, spend a few minutes taking inventory of your refrigerator, freezer, and pantry, and make a list of the staples that are running low. As you plan your menus for the week, jot down the items and ingredients that you need for your meals and recipes.

Don't forget to take your reading glasses with you. You'll need them to read the fine print of the nutrition labels. If you're a bargain shopper, a calculator can come in handy and save you a little brain-drain while you're comparing prices. If you're a coupon clipper, beware of the coupon trap. Some coupons might save you a little money, but they can also lead you into temptation, causing you to buy junk foods or other items that you would ordinarily avoid.

Saving money is great, but not when it's at the expense of your family's health. If you can't resist the lure of coupons, use them only for nonfood household items, like laundry detergent or furniture polish.

If you're the mother of small children, a trip to the grocery store can test the very limits of your patience and sanity. Make sure that you and your children are fed, watered, and well rested before you go. If your kids tend to get out of hand at the supermarket, taking just one child on each trip may be your best bet. Leaving your children at home with your spouse or a sitter is always tempting, but kids need lessons in shopping as much as they need lessons in math and reading. Selecting nutritious foods for a well-balanced diet is a skill that they'll need for the rest of their lives, and if you don't teach them, who will?

If you're the mother of a teen who would rather be caught parading around in an Elvis costume than be seen shopping with his mother, you'll have to be a little more creative. Schedule your shopping trip on the way home from ball practice, when you know your teen will be stuck with you and unable to escape. When older kids go shopping with you, ask them to help you find the ingredients for their favorite meals or allow them to choose nutritious items that they can snack on after school.

Try to make every trip to the supermarket a pleasant, stress-free experience for you and your kids by planning ahead. Before you go, allow your kids to make shopping suggestions so that you can discuss them while you're still at home. Do your bartering beforehand so that there won't be any bickering once you get to the store. Let your kids know that you'll be sticking to your shopping list and then stick to your guns. If your kids know the rules of the grocery shopping game ahead of time, they're more likely to abide by them, and shopping trips can become enjoyable, educational mother-child adventures.

The Produce Department

As soon as you've staked a claim on a shopping cart, head straight for the produce section. As the dietary director for your family, you'll want to encourage your kids to get at least five servings of fruits and veggies each day. If you don't buy these fruits and vegetables at the supermarket, the chances that you and your family will end up eating them are slim to none. It's almost impossible to ferret out five servings of fruits and veggies from a diet that contains mostly fast food and processed fare.

If you and your kids don't enjoy chopping, slicing, and dicing, you might as well bypass the whole, fresh-from-the-garden vegetables and head straight for the prewashed, precut varieties. These days, you can find just about every type of vegetable in a ready-to-eat state. If you don't find the prepared veggie you're looking for in the produce section, be sure to check the supermarket salad bar. It's usually stocked with chopped celery and onions, sliced peppers, cucumbers, and zucchini, as well as a few novelty items that you probably wouldn't take the time to fix yourself.

You can rustle up an entire salad from the salad bar, or you can find most salad fixings in ready-to-serve bags back at the produce department. Most supermarkets offer a wide variety of fresh, tasty salad greens as well as baby carrots, grape tomatoes, and florets of broccoli and cauliflower. In the time it takes to open the bags and toss the veggies together, you have a colorful, nutritious salad that the entire family will enjoy.

Many types of bagged vegetables make excellent additions to beef or chicken kabobs, and several lend themselves well to steaming and serving as side dishes. Prepared vegetables may cost a little more than the do-it-yourself varieties, but they can actually end up saving you money in the long run. After you trim away the stems, leaves, and stalks of whole vegetables, their prices may be comparable to those of the ready-to-eat varieties. If you never seem able to muster up the motivation to wash, slice, and dice the whole cauliflower heads and celery bunches that you bring home from the store, they're not really such a great bargain anyway. They're likely to end up in the garbage disposal, but only after spending a few weeks ripening to the extreme in the vegetable bin of your fridge. Because the prepared vegetables are more likely to wind up on the table than in the trashcan, they're a much better buy in the long run.

While you're in the produce section, be sure to pick up some fresh beans and peas. Snow peas, shelled lima beans, and precut string beans are quick and easy to fix, and they're an excellent source of protein and fiber. Corn on the cob is a family favorite, and it's a hassle-free addition to your main meal when you buy it fresh and free of shucks and silk. Don't forget to pick up some zucchini, squash, and eggplant. These veggies make colorful, flavorful side dishes, and all you have to do is wash, cut, steam, and serve. They also make nutritious additions to soups and pasta dishes.

Most kids love potatoes, so you'll want to have plenty on hand for baking and mashing. You can save yourself some time and work by choosing small, thin-skinned varieties. These can be boiled and baked without peeling, and they're great for adding to kabobs, roasts, vegetable dishes, and soups.

Since many of your recipes will call for peppers and onions, you'll want to make room for a few of each in your shopping cart. Not only do they add their own delectable, distinctive flavors, they also add vibrant colors. To increase the eye appeal of your dishes, choose red and yellow peppers in addition to green and look for red, yellow, and purple onions.

When you're finished shopping for vegetables, it's time to move on to the fruit. You really can't go wrong: the sweet tastes, bright colors, and fun textures of fruits make them fun-to-eat treats to most kids. Be sure to choose lots of fresh "finger" fruits like bananas, seedless grapes, apples, and oranges. These items travel well in lunchboxes, and because they don't require any preparation, they're great for kids to grab and eat on the run.

While they're in season, you'll want to choose fresh fruits that kids don't get a chance to eat every day. Apricots, blackberries, blueberries, plums, and cherries are tasty, nutritious treats that kids will be sure to eat and enjoy. Melons, like cantaloupe and honeydew, make fun fruit bowls for yogurt and cottage cheese. When they're cut into chunks and slices, they're great for adding to fruit salads or stacking on skewers for fruit kabobs.

Buying a variety of fresh berries is a good way to add fruit and flavor to breakfast foods, such as hot and cold cereals, pancakes, and waffles. They're also easy to use in the blender: just add a handful to a cup of vanilla yogurt for a nutritious fruit smoothie. Seedless grapes and bananas taste great fresh or frozen, and mashed bananas make a flavorful, low-calorie extender for peanut butter.

If preparing whole fruit seems too labor-intensive and makes you weary just thinking about it, don't hesitate to buy ready-to-eat fruit in plastic bags and containers. Without the rinds, skins, and seeds, they may not be such a bad buy. If you don't see what you're looking for in the produce department, try the salad bar. You can usually find wedges of pineapple and seedless watermelon, sliced kiwi and strawberries, and a variety of brightly colored melon balls.

You can get the most for your produce dollar by choosing fruits and vegetables that have the most to offer in the way of nutrition. Although all fruits and vegetables are excellent sources of fiber, some supply more vitamins and minerals than others. In most cases, the darker-colored fruits, such as apricots, oranges, and strawberries, are better sources of nutrients than their lighter-colored counterparts, such as apples and pears, which are pale beneath their vibrant skins. The same is true for darker-colored vegetables. Broccoli, Brussels sprouts, carrots, spinach, and sweet potatoes contain more vitamins and minerals than cucumbers, celery, and iceberg lettuce.

While you're in the produce department, don't forget to pick up a variety of fresh, unsalted nuts. Pecans, walnuts, hazelnuts, and Brazil nuts are loaded with protein, and a serving of nuts can replace a serving of meat in a healthy, well-balanced diet. While they're typically rather high in fat, the fat they contain is that of the heart-healthy variety. Nuts are crunchy, satisfying, and filling, making them an excellent caloric investment.

In some supermarkets, a selection of dried fruit can be found in the produce department. You'll want to pick up a bag or two for your kids to snack on, either alone or as a tasty, nutritious addition to homemade trail mixes. When preparing trail mixes, however, note that not all dried fruits are created equal. Dried fruits like prunes, pineapples, pears, raisins, and apples are excellent choices; they're a fat-free, fiber-rich source of high-energy nutrients. Watch out for the "dried" bananas. They're often fried and can contain as many as 16 grams of fat in a single two-thirds cup serving.

The Meat Department

When you've loaded your shopping cart with all the fruits and veggies you need, it's time to head to the meat department.

Fresh Meat

Meats of all types are an excellent source of protein, iron, and other minerals, but like all animal products, they also contain fat and cholesterol. The amount of fat and cholesterol in each serving of meat depends largely on the cut and the source. Beef, pork, and lamb are typically high in fat, but any cut of these meats that contains the word "loin" or "round" in its name is a lean cut. Choosing the leanest cuts of beef, pork, and lamb you can find will significantly lower the amount of fat you get from each serving. Beef round steak, beef loin tip, sirloin steak, and pork and lamb loin chops are quite a bit lower in fat than other cuts. When you're preparing these types of meat at home, be sure to trim all visible fat before cooking and drain the grease when you're finished.

Most working moms rely on ground beef for making quick and easy recipes. Although it tends to be a little higher in fat than other types of beef, it's not necessary to give it up altogether. Just be sure to use the leanest ground beef you can buy. Ground round is lower in fat than ground chuck, which is lower in fat than meat that is simply labeled "ground beef." Lean ground beef is a little more expensive per pound than regular ground beef, but since you'll have less fat to drain after cooking it, you'll actually end up with more meat for your money.

You can reduce the fat content of any type of ground beef after cooking it by draining it well and patting it with paper towels to remove as much fat as possible. If you're willing to go the extra mile, you can even place the cooked meat in a colander and rinse it with hot water. After draining it and patting it dry, it will be just as tasty, but much lower in fat and calories.

When a recipe calls for cooked ground beef, make sure that each serving contains no more than 3 ounces of meat. In most cases, you can use a little less meat and a little more of something else that contains less fat. Spaghetti sauce can be bulked up and flavored with whole tomatoes, mushrooms, and other chopped vegetables in place of meat. Chili tastes just as delicious when you use less meat and more beans. Legumes like dried beans and peas are good alternative sources of protein, and they have a lot less fat, calories, and cholesterol than meat.

Ground turkey and chicken are good choices, as long as the skin is removed and they don't contain added fat. Before you make room for them in your shopping cart, check the nutrition labels for fat and calorie content and compare them to the leanest ground beef available.

Soy crumbles are a nutritious substitute for cooked ground beef, and you probably won't be able to tell the difference in seasoned foods like chili, tacos, and spaghetti sauce. Using the soy substitute will save your family some extra fat, and because you don't have to cook it, it will save you time in preparation and cleanup. While soy substitutes are occasionally stocked in the meat department, you might also find them in the produce department or frozen foods aisle.

To lower the fat and cholesterol content of your family's diet, try serving poultry and fish in place of red meat at least a couple of nights a week. Whether you're buying meat, poultry, or fish, remember that 3 cooked ounces is the recommended portion size, which is about the size of a deck of cards. Unless you plan to double your recipes and save the extra for later, try to buy packages of meat that contain just enough to provide a single serving for each member of your family. When there aren't any leftovers, you and your kids won't be tempted to take second helpings or eat more than you planned.

If you're not crazy about skinning and deboning poultry products, be sure to buy items like boneless, skinless chicken and turkey breasts. They cost a little more per pound than the whole-bird products, but the time and energy they save is well worth the extra price. If you buy whole birds, remember that the skin contains most of the fat and be sure to remove it before cooking. White meat is lower in fat and calories than dark meat, but dark meat is richer in iron.

With each trip to the supermarket, you're likely to see new convenience products in the meat department. You can now find precooked roast beef, beef tips, pork roast, and chicken. Although these convenience items may contain slightly more fat per serving than those you prepare yourself, they usually contain a lot less fat and fewer calories than fast food meals. For really quick and easy meals at home, it's hard to beat items like precooked and seasoned strips or chunks of chicken and turkey. They're great for adding to salads, stir-fry dishes, fajitas, and burritos.

Packaged Meats

These days, you can find a wide variety of lean and reduced-fat packaged meats and deli cuts in your supermarket's meat department. Several manufacturers offer deli meats like ham, turkey, and roast beef in a "97 percent fat free" variety. These meats are great for making sandwiches and snacks.

Limit your use of regular processed meats, which tend to be high in fat and sodium. Summer sausage, salami, and pepperoni typically contain about 15 to 20 grams of fat per serving. Avoid the high-fat "regular" hot dogs and bologna and opt for the low-fat or reduced-fat versions of these family favorites. A single slice of regular bologna packs about 22 grams of fat, 240 calories, and 810 milligrams of sodium, so you'll want to steer clear of it whenever you can, opting instead for the low-fat or reduced-fat versions. Because manufacturers and food processors use different recipes and ingredients in their products, you and your family may find some fat-free renditions of the real things more appealing than others. If you're not crazy about the first brand you choose, be sure to try another one before you give up and go back to the full-fat variety.

When you're buying packaged or processed meat, you can't always be sure that products made with turkey or chicken are lower in fat than the traditional products. Some manufacturers use added fat or poultry skins in their recipes. Be sure to read and compare nutrition labels before you buy.

Your kids will probably fall hook, line, and sinker for packaged mini-meals like Lunchables and Snackables, but be sure to check the nutrition labels before you cave in to their requests. These types of foods may be convenient and fun for kids to eat, but they're packed with fat, calories, and sodium. A single serving of Lunchables Nachos, for example, has 570 calories, 29 grams of fat, and 1,160 milligrams of sodium.

If you're watching your cholesterol count, you'll want to limit your use of organ meats, such as liver, kidneys, and brains. If you can't resist sausage and bacon, it's not a crime to eat them on occasion, but their high fat content should prohibit them from being breakfast staples. A single 2-ounce serving of pork sausage has 22 grams of fat and about 240 calories. Rather than making these high-fat meats the main course of the meal, try incorporating them into recipes. You can still enjoy their rich flavor and avoid some of the caloric consequences. With 35 calories and 2.5 grams of fat per serving, turkey bacon is a better choice than the traditional pork varieties, which usually contain 90 calories and 7 grams of fat in a single serving.

The Dairy Case

In most supermarkets, the meat department is adjacent to the dairy case, where you'll find a huge selection of nutritious and delicious foods. Almost every dairy product imaginable now comes in a fat-free or reduced-fat variety. If you're watching your weight, they're much better for you, and they taste just as good as the regular items. Use "lite" or low-fat dairy products every chance you get. You'll still get plenty of beneficial nutrients and good taste, but not fat. Try the reduced-fat or low-fat versions of dairy foods like cheese, sour cream, cream cheese, cottage cheese, and yogurt. While low-fat yogurt has only around 2 grams of fat per serving, whole-milk yogurt has about 7 grams per serving. Choosing fat-free cheeses over the regular varieties can save you around 10 grams of fat per serving. Most fat-free dairy products can be used in almost any recipe as a substitute for the higher-fat varieties. Drinking fat-free milk is an excellent way for older kids and adults to get the calcium they need without getting too much fat.

Although kids under two need whole milk and whole-milk dairy products, you can buy skim or fat-free milk for yourself and your older children. While skim milk offers just 2 grams of fat per serving, whole milk provides 16 grams. If your family is accustomed to drinking whole milk, it may take a while for them to get used to the fat-free or skim variety. You can ease the transition by mixing equal parts of whole milk and fat-free milk and then gradually reducing the proportion of whole milk until you eliminate it completely.

If your family seems unable to stomach the fat-free milk, you might have better luck getting them to drink the 1 percent or 2 percent varieties. You can still use fat-free milk in your recipes, and no one will even know the difference.

When choosing flavored yogurts for snacks, you might want to buy the ones that are sweetened with sugar substitutes and those that are low in fat or fat free. Individual pudding and gelatin cups are great to keep on hand for quick snacks and for packing in lunchboxes. Look for the low-fat or fat-free puddings and avoid the high-fat cheesecakes, custards, and similar treats. For a little extra nutrition and fiber, choose gelatin cups with added chunks of fruit. Individually wrapped packages of string cheese are a fun way for kids to get the calcium that their growing bodies need.

You can find egg substitutes in the dairy case at your supermarket. Try using them in your recipes to reduce their fat and cholesterol content. They're easy to use and mess-free, and you won't be able to taste the difference.

Use sticks of margarine and real butter only when required in recipes. Remember, products that are liquid at room temperature contain less saturated fat than solid ones. For this reason, liquid squeeze margarine is a better choice than soft margarine in tubs, which in turn is a better choice than the solid margarine in sticks. Butter-flavored sprays from the dairy case add a nice touch to vegetables, popcorn, and bread without adding much fat. For cooking, use nonstick vegetable sprays or small amounts of canola or olive oil.

Canned biscuits, rolls, and breadsticks all come in tasty low-fat and reduced-fat versions. Check out the recommended serving sizes before you buy them. A "grand"-sized biscuit is usually twice the size of a regular biscuit, with twice the calories and fat. Look for canned biscuits in whole-wheat or other whole-grain varieties to add nutrients and fiber to your family's diet. While you're in the dairy case, be sure to pick up some low-fat pizza crusts and tortillas. They're great for using in quick and easy recipes, and kids love eating them.

When choosing prepared fruit drinks from the dairy case, look for those that contain 100 percent fruit juice. If a fruit beverage is labeled "drink," "ade," or "cocktail," it contains flavored sugar-water with just a splash of fruit juice. Manufacturers of fruit drinks are required to list the products' ingredients on the packages, as well as the percentage fruit juice they contain. Be sure to check the label before you add a fruit drink to your shopping cart. Fruit juices are far better than sodas, but they're still full of natural sugars, and they're high in calories and low in fiber. It's fine to allow kids to have a serving of fruit juice every day, but giving them a glass of water and a piece of whole fruit is a much more nutritious and filling way for them to meet their daily requirements for fluids, fiber, vitamins, and minerals.

Frozen Foods Section

Most working moms with roomy freezers rely heavily on items from the frozen foods section of their grocery stores. You can find dozens of nutritious, delicious meals and ingredients for recipes hidden among the high fat, calorie-laden convenience foods.

Frozen vegetables are excellent for adding to recipes, and you can find more than just corn, carrots, and peas. Mixtures of stir-fry, Southwestern, and Oriental vegetables add just the right touch to your entrees and can save you hours of shopping and chopping time. In the winter months, when many fresh vegetables are out of season or outrageously expensive, frozen vegetables are a good substitute for the real thing. You can buy ready-to-eat corn on the cob, broccoli and cauliflower florets, Brussels sprouts, beans, and peas in several varieties. Most packaged, frozen vegetables are rich in fiber and low in calories and contain no added fat or cholesterol, so you can use them liberally at every meal.

Frozen fruits are easy and fun to use, but be on the lookout for added sugar. Most food manufacturers cook berries with sugar before freezing them. If you look hard enough, you'll probably be able to find a few items that don't include added sugar. The frozen fruit salad mixes are always popular. Kids love the melon balls, grapes, and strawberries, especially when they're served partially frozen.

While the prepared entrees and side dishes in the frozen food section look appetizing and effortless, they're usually loaded with fat, sodium, and calories. If you want to buy frozen dinners for your family every now and then, be sure to choose the ones geared toward dieters. Weight Watchers, Lean Cuisine, and Healthy Choice make dozens of tasty dishes that typically have fewer than 8 grams of fat and no more than 350 calories per serving.

You can now find a huge selection of health-wrecking junk food in your grocer's freezer case, including fried, frozen egg rolls, pizza bites and bagels, tater tots, and onion rings. Your kids will find them very appealing, but your best bet is to steer clear of them altogether. Most of these foods have very little to offer in the way of nutrition, and your kids would probably be better off eating the cardboard packages than the foods themselves.

Drag your kids away from the fried, frozen junk foods and offer them frozen fruit and dairy treats instead. These are foods that your kids will love, and ones that you won't mind them eating. Encourage your kids to choose frozen yogurt with fruit instead of rich, chocolate-filled ice cream and look for frozen fruit juice products instead of the artificially flavored, sugar-packed Popsicles. Products like Minute Maid 90 Percent Fruit Bars are tasty, low-calorie, fat-free alternatives that kids will go for. Pay close attention to the nutrition labels of novelty ice cream treats. Items like M&M Ice Cream Cones look oh-so-tempting, but they pack 230 calories and 11 grams of fat in a single serving.

You can make frozen yogurt with fruit even more fun to eat by serving it in brightly colored ice cream cups and sugar cones. Sugar cones are fat free, and each one contains only 60 calories, while green, pink, and brown "rainbow" ice cream cups have just 20 calories and contain no fat.

The freezer cases in modern-day supermarkets have expanded to accommodate a wide variety of new and more convenient breakfast foods. Frozen waffles are easy for kids to fix and fun to eat, and the fat-free varieties are good investments. Two plain Eggo Fat Free Waffles have no fat and just 120 calories per serving. If you can talk your kids into leaving off the butter and sugary syrup and top them with fruit instead, they can be a part of a nutritious breakfast. Regular waffles aren't always such a great selection. Two Eggo Homestyle Waffles contain 7 grams of fat and 190 calories. As your kids pile on butter and syrup, the caloric content of their breakfast climbs. Topping two regular waffles with a couple of tablespoons of butter and a quarter cup of syrup makes breakfast a 400-calorie affair, with about 25 grams of fat to boot.

The makers of Toaster Strudels have hit kids hard with cool television commercials, but the products themselves are less than ideal. With lots of sugar and 10 grams of fat per serving, a Cream Cheese and Strawberry Pastry isn't all that cool. Whatever you do, don't fall for the breakfast equivalents of TV dinners; most of them are swimming in fat, cholesterol, and sodium. Swanson's Great Starts Scrambled Eggs and Sausage packs 27 grams of fat, 330 milligrams of cholesterol, and 670 milligrams of sodium into a single serving. Eating this type of breakfast isn't really such a great way to start your morning after all.

Watch out for frozen breads and biscuits; they often contain lots of added fat and calories. Pillsbury Home Baked Classics biscuits have 180 calories, 9 grams of fat, and 570 milligrams of cholesterol tucked into each one. Frozen bagels and English muffins are excellent choices for breakfast, and they're great for making low-fat snacks like miniature pizzas and sandwiches. Look for the whole-wheat varieties; they offer a little more in the way of nutrition and fiber than the refined products.

Canned Foods

In the winter months, a wide selection of fresh fruits and vegetables will be a little harder to come by, so you'll probably end up choosing canned fruits and vegetables from time to time. Canned fruits contain less fiber and fewer vitamins and minerals than fresh fruits, but they'll certainly do in a pinch. Be sure to choose fruits canned in "lite" syrup or fruit juice whenever possible; they have a lot less sugar and calories than those prepared with heavy syrup. Kids are usually happy to eat the old standbys, like peaches, fruit cocktail, pears, and pineapples, but it's always fun for them to experiment with new tastes and textures. Many exotic fruits are available in cans, like tiny mandarin oranges, kiwi, and mango.

Most kids love applesauce, but make sure to choose brands with no added sugar. Applesauce is now available with many added flavors, like watermelon, blueberry, and cinnamon. The bright blue, green, and red colors make them even more appealing to kids. Individual servings of applesauce or fruit cups with light syrup make great additions to school lunches or after-school snacks.

Almost every type of vegetable imaginable can be found in a can. These days, you can buy most canned vegetables with no added salt, an option that can significantly reduce your family's sodium intake. If your favorite canned vegetables aren't available in a no-added-salt version, you can place them in a strainer and rinse them with water before you prepare them.

Beans are some of your best buys in the canned food section of your supermarket. Because they're packed with protein, a serving of many types of beans can replace a serving of meat. Most varieties are high in fiber and rich in nutrients. Be sure to stock up on plenty of black-eyed peas, kidney beans, garbanzo beans (chickpeas), lima beans, and green peas. Baked beans aren't as nutritious as other varieties of beans, but those labeled "vegetarian style" often have less fat and fewer calories than the meat-flavored versions.

While you're in the canned food section of your grocery store, be sure to pick up plenty of canned tomato products to use in your favorite recipes. Canned tomato paste, tomato sauce, and whole and diced tomatoes are good plant sources of iron, and they're packed with vitamins. Processed tomato products are also rich in lycopenes, which have been shown to reduce the risk of several types of cancer.

If you've got the time and energy to make tomato-based sauces from scratch, then by all means go for it. If you're pressed for time, be sure to pick up some ready-made spaghetti sauce and pizza sauce. Most manufacturers offer reduced-fat versions, and they're great to have on hand to use in recipes. Look for meatless varieties that are made with vegetable chunks to help your kids pack more veggies into their diets.

Canned soups are indispensable in dozens of quick, convenient meals or recipes. Fortunately, most varieties are now available in low-fat or reduced-calorie versions. Choosing low-fat cream-based soups instead of the regular ones can end up saving you 4 or 5 grams of fat and 35 to 50 calories per serving. When you're serving soup as a meal or snack, your best bet is to choose vegetable and bean soups rather than the creamy varieties, which are almost always higher in fat.

Most kids love ramen noodle soups, but they probably have a lot more fat than you think. One package of ramen noodles typically contains two servings, and each serving packs 8 grams of fat and a whopping 800 milligrams of sodium. Eating the noodles every now and then isn't going to kill your kids, but be sure to compare nutrition labels before you buy them and choose the baked versions rather than those that are fried.

Most canned pastas, like ravioli or spaghetti with tomato sauce, are fine for kids to snack on from time to time. The meatless varieties are typically lower in fat and calories than those prepared with meat, and many varieties now come in reduced-fat versions.

Canned tuna fish is an excellent source of high-quality protein. To cut down on unwanted fat, choose tuna that is packed in water rather than oil. Some brands of tuna now come packaged in pouches with no added moisture, eliminating the hassle and mess of draining. Tuna packed in pouches is much easier to use in recipes or to enjoy eating right out of the package.

You can also find skinless, boneless salmon in pouches, and the tasty, nutritious fish can be used in place of tuna in most recipes. Both tuna and salmon are excellent sources of protein, and because they're rich in omega-3 fatty acids, they're an important addition to a heart-healthy diet.

Grains and Pasta Aisle

You'll find plenty of nutritious items in this section of the supermarket. Many types of rice and pasta are fortified with extra vitamins and minerals. Be sure to stock up on plenty of whole grains like brown rice and barley to serve with your main courses or add to soups and other recipes. Most kids love pasta, and you can find a wide variety of interesting colors, shapes, and sizes that make them even more fun to eat. You can usually find pasta made from whole wheat, spinach, and other nutritious ingredients.

Baked Goods Section

While there are plenty of wholesome, nutritious items in this section, they're usually surrounded by products that are loaded with fat and sugar. Strategically placed fresh doughnuts, pastries, cakes, and pies will catch your eye, but there's no room for these types of foods in your shopping cart. To get the most nutrition for your money, choose whole-grain breads instead of refined white breads. You'll dramatically increase the amount of fiber, vitamins, and minerals your kids get when they eat toast or sandwiches. Buy a variety of fun, nutritious breads, such as whole-wheat pita pockets for stuffing, whole-wheat bagels and English muffins for making mini-pizzas and snacks, and whole-grain sub rolls and buns for making sandwiches.

Breakfast Foods Aisle

You'll want to get a firm grip on your kids before you journey through this aisle. Kids are bombarded with television advertisements for sugary breakfast cereals that are virtually fiber free, artificially flavored and colored, and loaded with preservatives and additives. It's not a crime to allow your kids to pick a cool new cereal every now and then, even if it's not a nutritional superstar. Even the "worst" cereals are made better with a serving of lowfat milk, and they're still far superior nutritionally to many other traditional high-fat breakfast foods, such as doughnuts and sweet rolls.

Be sure to check the nutrition labels, starting with the sugar content. Some breakfast cereals, especially those made for children, are 35 to 50 percent sugar by weight. You might as well feed your kids a couple of chocolate chip cookies or a slice of cake for breakfast. Look for cereals that have fewer than 6 to 9 grams of sugar per serving, and those that offer at least a couple of grams of fiber.

To make sure that your kids are getting the most from the morning meal, look for words like "whole-grain" before ingredients like rice, corn, or barley on the box. This means that they're probably a reasonable source of complex carbohydrates and fiber.

Most cereals, even those that are packed with sugar, are naturally low in fat, with granola cereals and those containing coconut being the exceptions. These cereals can contain around 8 grams of fat in a single 1-ounce serving. They may not be as bad as they look on first glance, as they typically provide lots of fiber. The fat contained in many of these cereals is often unsaturated fat, which isn't as detrimental as fat of the saturated variety.

You can find a wide variety of breakfast pastries and sugar-sweetened cereal bars in the breakfast aisle of the supermarket. These are typically fortified with lots of vitamins and minerals, but they're still high in sugar and low in fiber. If you're looking for something for kids to eat on the run, fruit-filled fiber bars are better choices. Individual packages of hot cereals, like oatmeal and cream of wheat, are nutritionally sound breakfast choices, and they're as easy to make as heating a cup of water in the microwave. Fun flavors like strawberry, peach, and cinnamon raisin make them even more tempting for kids to eat.

Snack Foods Aisle

By the time you get around to the snack food aisle, your shopping cart should be almost full of wholesome, nutritious items, and it's just as well. The snack food aisle is one of the danger zones of your grocery store, and you'll need to pass through it in a state of alert. Most selections in this section are packed with fat, cholesterol, sugar, salt, and calories. You can dramatically limit these nutritional bad guys in your family's diet by choosing snacks that are fat free or at least low in fat. Your best buys are snacks that are baked rather than fried. Choose baked chips, pretzels, and flavored rice cakes instead of chips and crackers fried in oil.

Fat-free chips may contain the fat substitute Olestra, which is okay for your kids to eat every now and then, but not on a regular basis. Overzealous consumption of Olestra-containing snacks can lead to stomach cramping and diarrhea and may even result in the loss of fat-soluble vitamins from the body.

Watch out for the single-serving convenience packages of chips and dip. A package of Frito Lay Corn Chips and Chili Cheese Dip contains 10 grams of fat, while Doritos Nacho Cheesier Dip and Chips serves up a whopping 32 grams of fat, 610 calories, and an incredible 1,060 milligrams of sodium.

Although the ready-to-snack-on flavored popcorns might sound like a low-fat food, they're not. A single serving of popcorn seasoned with white cheddar cheese packs around 9 grams of fat. If your kids enjoy snacking on popcorn, buy the type that you make in the microwave and choose the low-fat versions instead of the regular varieties.

Beverage Aisle

When you get to the soda section of your supermarket, just keep on moving till you find the fruit juices and bottled water. If you don't want your kids drinking soft drinks, don't put them into your shopping cart. Sports drinks really aren't any better than other soft drinks. If your kids are athletes who exercise strenuously for more than an hour a day, they might actually need the replacement electrolytes contained in sports drinks. For most other kids, they're too high in sugar to drink on a regular basis.

Make it a family policy not to bring sodas, sugar-sweetened drinks, or flavored drink mixes in your home. They have nothing to offer but calories and cavities, and your kids will get plenty of these beverages away from home.

If you need bottled or boxed beverages to take on road trips or pack in lunches, choose 100 percent fruit juice or bottled water. When you're buying bottled water for your kids, you might want to choose the brands that contain fluoride to help protect their teeth from cavities.

Condiments

You'll want to stock up on a wide assortment of seasonings to add extra flavor to your meals without a lot of extra work. Many condiments are fairly benign, but just as many are loaded with fat, sodium, and sugar. When you're choosing items that are typically high in salt, like ketchup and soy sauce, opt for the low-sodium versions. Since most varieties of mustard are fat free and low in salt and fat, you're pretty safe putting them in your shopping cart.

Regular mayonnaise, salad dressings, and dips typically contain around 9 grams of fat per teaspoon, so you'll definitely want to buy the fat-free renditions to use in recipes and on salads and sandwiches. Pickles and relishes are great to use to jazz up salads and sandwiches, and most varieties are fat free and low in calories. If you're watching your sodium intake, you'll want to use them sparingly, because most types are prepared with lots of salt. Be sure to pick up a few jars of salsa to use for nutritious, low-fat dipping and to have on hand to add to recipes.

In this section of your supermarket, you'll probably be able to find packaged seasoning mixes for soups, dips, and main meals, such as meatloaf, tacos, and chili. Buying these packages is a lot less expensive than buying the individual containers of all the spices they contain, and they can make life in the kitchen a lot easier.

Peanut butter and jelly are usually stocked in the condiment section of the supermarket, and if your kids love them, you'll want to pick up some of each.

While regular peanut butter usually provides about 17 grams of fat in each 2-tablespoon serving, the reduced-fat varieties contain around 11 grams of fat, which is still relatively high. Peanut butter is an excellent source of kid-friendly protein, so you won't want to nix it completely. Just make sure your kids know not to slather it two inches thick on their sandwiches and crackers. If you want to add flavor and bulk to peanut butter without adding extra fat, try mixing a couple of tablespoons with mashed bananas.

Most jams and jellies are fat free, but they're loaded with sugar. You can reduce the number of calories your kids get per serving by choosing products that are made from whole fruit with no added sugar. Stay away from the prepackaged snacks with crackers, peanut butter, and jelly. Each serving contains over 400 calories and 20 grams of fat.

Ketchup, mustard, and low-fat squeeze margarine now come in a variety of cool colors, like green, pink, and purple. You might want to invest in a bottle or two so that your kids can dress up their meals with colorful designs. They'll have a lot of fun grossing out their parents by making and eating weird-colored foods.

Nonfood Items

If you're planning to make quick and easy dinners at home, you'll need a few nonfood staples. It's a good idea to have plenty of oven browning bags on hand for baking chicken and roasting meats and vegetables. Lining your baking sheets and dishes with aluminum foil helps seal in the flavor of baked foods and makes clean-up a lot easier. Don't forget to buy paper bags for lunches and pint-size plastic bags for making up individual homemade snack packs with nutritious items like fruits, vegetables, or trail mix.

Buy a few utensils and tools that kids can use to help you out in the kitchen, like cookie cutters, potato mashers, and handheld veggie choppers. You can always find grated cheese at the supermarket, but you might want to buy a cheese grater anyway, if for no other reason than its kid appeal and entertainment value. While you're handling the riskier kitchen tools and appliances, like sharp knives and hot ovens, kids can safely take part in meal preparation by grating cheese and shredding and chopping vegetables.

Kids love to decorate just about anything, including their food. While you're shopping, buy a couple of inexpensive saltshakers and fill each one with powdered sugar, cinnamon, and several colors of sugar sprinkles. Your kids can use them to decorate their toast, breakfast cereal, oatmeal, and just about anything else. Once kids get involved in adding their own unique designs to their meals, they're much more likely to eat them.

While you're shopping, pick up an empty plastic squeeze bottle. You can fill it with low-fat yogurt at home so that kids can have fun squirting tasty, calcium-rich yogurt onto their oatmeal or fruit chunks.

Be sure to buy some wooden skewer sticks so that kids can make and eat their own fruit and veggie kabobs. Colored toothpicks are also good to have on hand. Kids can use them like Tinker Toys, connecting them with chunks of fruit and vegetables to build their own deliciously edible figures and structures.

If you don't have a Crock-Pot or other slow cooker, now is a good time to make the investment. You and your kids will have fun making easy, nutritious meals in it. It only takes a few minutes to chop up some fresh vegetables and place them in the slow cooker with chicken, beef, and a can of soup or broth. Just turn the cooker on in the morning before you leave for work and school, and you'll return home to a delicious aroma and a tasty, wholesome meal.

Don't forget to buy a cooler or an insulated bag for your car. You can keep it stocked with bottled water and fruit juices, as well as fruit cups, yogurt, vegetables, and other nutritious finger foods. Having tasty snacks on hand in the car will keep your kids satisfied and make it easier for you to pass up the drive-through window at your favorite fast food restaurant.

Chapter 10

Packing the Healthy Lunchbox

Each day in the United States, about 25 million children in over 95,000 schools eat lunches provided through the National School Lunch Program (NSLP). All of these lunches must meet the Dietary Guidelines for Americans and other nutritional standards, which recommend that no more than 30 percent of the meals' calories come from fat. The meals served must provide a third of a child's daily calories and other nutrients.

While school lunches must meet federal nutrition requirements, local school officials still have the final say about what foods will be served and how they will be prepared. A recent study conducted by the U.S. Department of Agriculture (USDA) showed that during the 1990s, fat content of school lunches declined dramatically, while offerings of fruits and vegetables increased. Although meals served in school cafeterias are getting better, they're still far from ideal—especially in terms of taste and kid appeal. Dwindling school budgets dramatically impact the taste and quality of the meals offered. In many cases, foods used in the NSLP are dictated by surplus supplies of pork, beef, cheese, and other products provided to schools by the USDA.

Even if the lunches served up by the school cafeteria are nutritious, there's still the problem of getting kids to eat them. If your child isn't crazy about cafeteria-style food, he may shun the lunch line and head straight for a vending machine, fast food counter, or snack bar, options that are popping up in a growing number of school cafeterias.

To help deliver your child from the temptation of purchasing sugary, high-fat junk food and fast food, your best bet might be to send your child to school with a lunchbox filled with nutritious fare instead of a pocketful of spending money.

Before packing a boxed lunch, you'll need a few simple items. Allow your child to pick out a lunchbox or small cooler that she'll be willing to carry to school each day. Make sure that you buy a small freezer pack to keep the food inside cold and safe to eat.

Most school cafeterias now have microwave ovens that are accessible to students. If you want your child to eat a hot meal, simply pack the ingredients in microwave-safe containers so he'll be able to heat them up before eating them.

If your child will drink milk with her meal, she can buy it in the cafeteria at lunchtime. If she doesn't like milk or can't tolerate it, you may have to include a drink in her lunchbox. Bottled water is always an excellent choice, but be sure to include a carton of fruit or vegetable juice every now and then to give her a little variety.

Making a nutritious, fun-to-eat lunch for your child each day doesn't have to be complicated. You don't have to spend a lot of time in the kitchen cooking up culinary wonders: most kids enjoy simple fare. What they really love is opening up their creative minds when they open up their lunchboxes. Just adding a few simple touches can spice up a nutritious lunch with a little mystery, surprise, or challenge.

All of the menus below are rich in vitamins, minerals, and fiber and offer fewer than 10 grams of fat. Each meal includes at least one food from four of the five basic food groups: grain, fruit, vegetable, and meat and protein. Many of them contain a food from the dairy group, but for those that don't, a carton of low-fat milk will complete the nutritional picture.

Missing from each lunch are high-fat, sugary desserts. By the time kids are actually seated at the lunch table in the school cafeteria, they usually have just about fifteen minutes to spend eating. Many children, especially those that are slow eaters, will run out of time before finishing their meals. By leaving junk food out of her lunchbox, you'll be sure that your child isn't passing over the more nutritious items and heading straight for the "treat."

You don't have to limit yourself to the menus listed here—these are just a few suggestions to help get you started. Ask your child to help you create theme lunches or special meals with the foods and ingredients that she likes best. It only takes a few simple suggestions from Mom to fire up a child's imagination and make lunch an eating adventure.

Action Plan

✔ **Tuck some TLC into your child's lunch.** A short note from you with a few words of love or encouragement makes lunchboxes more fun to open.

✔ **Speak your mind.** If you're concerned about the ready availability of snacks and sodas on your child's school campus, let school officials know. Write a letter to the school board or attend PTA meetings and voice your opinions.

✔ **Take a clue from what your kids are learning in school.** If they're studying state history, for example, create for them a state-themed menu, which will add color and fun to their lunch as well as their studies.

✔ **Don't be shy with leftovers from dinner.** While kids do need variety, a second helping from a nutritious and delicious meal every now and then will surely brighten their lunchbox—especially if the meal was a hit

✔ **Practice what you preach.** Take your own healthy packed lunch with you to work.

Crazy Eights

8	whole-wheat crackers
8	ham squares (2 slices low-fat ham, cut into quarters)
8	cheese squares (2 slices fat-free cheese, cut into quarters)
8	strawberries
8	baby carrots
8	celery sticks (2 stalks celery, cut into quarters)
8	animal crackers or 2 graham crackers divided into 8 pieces

Tic Tac Toe

½	whole-wheat pita stuffed with low-fat chicken salad
¼	cup raisins
¾	cup crunchy cereal
1	cup broccoli and cauliflower florets
¼	cup fat-free dressing for dip

On a 3" x 5" index card or piece of paper, draw tic-tac-toe grids. Use raisins and cereal pieces for Xs and Os.

Safari Lunch

1	safari sub sandwich: whole-wheat bun, low-fat deli meat and fat-free cheese, lettuce, and tomato
1	"jungle fruit" banana
½	cup "quicksand" low-fat chocolate pudding
1	cup "rainforest" broccoli and cauliflower florets
¼	cup low-fat dressing for dip
15	"jungle animals" animal crackers

Guess What?

1 sandwich made with whole-wheat bread and low-fat deli meat
¼ cup low-fat cheese chunks
1 small orange, cut into sections or sliced
½ cup strawberries
½ cup broccoli florets
8 baby carrots

Place the sandwich in a clear plastic bag, so your child can eat it while she works on the riddles and learns a little about nutrition. Wrap remaining lunch items in aluminum foil. Cut a 3" x 5" index card into squares and write riddles on them before taping to the appropriate aluminum-wrapped food item. You can make the clues easier or more difficult depending on your child's age.

Orange: I am a round, orange fruit that grows in warm climates. I am rich in vitamin C and often used to make a breakfast juice. What am I?
Strawberries: I am a small, red fruit used to make jams and jellies. What am I?
Broccoli: I am a green vegetable that grows in bunches. I am a good source of fiber. What am I?
Carrots: I am an orange vegetable that grows underground. Rabbits love me. What am I?
Cheese: I am made from milk and am a good source of calcium. My color is orange. What am I?

Favorite Baseball (or other sport) Team Lunch

1 whole-wheat hot dog bun
1 all-beef, low-sodium hot dog
1 cup popped popcorn
   Baseballs (½ cup melon balls or ¼ cup raisins)
   Baseball bats (1 cup baby carrots or celery or carrot sticks)

Tuck a few baseball cards into your child's lunchbox, or a drawing of the team logo or mascot. (You can draw it yourself or print it from the website of your child's favorite team.)

Seaside Lunch

1	peanut butter and "jellyfish" sandwich
⅓	cup fish-shaped crackers
	Sand dollar apple slices
⅓	cup fish-shaped gummy treats
½	cup broccoli florets (palm trees)
	Sand pail and shovel (cup of low-fat yogurt and plastic spoon)

In your child's lunchbox, place a picture of your family at the beach and a few of the seashells you collected while you were there. She'll enjoy reminiscing or telling her friends about her vacation while she eats her lunch.

Pirate's Treasure

1	Treasure chest of chicken (square plastic container with baked chicken fingers)
½	cup golden carrot "coins"
¼	cup yogurt covered raisin "pearls"
½	cup low-fat chocolate or vanilla "Pirate" pudding
2	"walk the plank" whole-wheat breadsticks

Add a few "treasures" to your child's lunch box, like a small toy, a few coins, or a treasure map that leads to a hidden surprise that he can search for at home after school.

Alphabet Lunch

1	Pizza (½ English muffin or bagel topped with pizza sauce and cheese)
1	ounce pretzels
1	small peach or plum
1	small green pepper, sliced
½	cup low-fat pudding

Pack foods that all begin with the same letter of the alphabet. Include a small wrapped toy or prize for your child to open after she guesses the letter that inspired her lunch.

Skewer Lunch

1   Wooden skewer with chunks of low-fat ham, and cheese

1   Wooden skewer with grape tomatoes, green peppers, and cauliflower florets

1   Wooden skewer with chunks of pineapple, grapes, melon, and strawberries

1   cup low-fat yogurt for fruit dip

¼   cup low-fat dressing for veggie dip

8   whole-wheat crackers

After loading skewers, you might want to cut off the pointed ends to prevent accidental injury to your child and his lunchmates.

Deli Lunch

   Lettuce leaves

   Tomato slices

1   3-ounce serving sliced low-fat deli meat

1   slice low-fat cheese

1   Whole-wheat submarine sandwich roll

1   Sliced pickles, olives, or green peppers

1   cup low-fat fruit yogurt

Kids love to eat their own creations. By packaging each ingredient separately, you allow your child to have fun building and eating his own special sandwich.

Salad Bar Lunch

   Shredded spinach leaves

¼   cup low-fat ham chunks

¼   cup shredded low-fat cheese

¼   cup each grape tomatoes, sliced carrots, and broccoli or cauliflower florets

¼   cup fat-free salad dressing

¼   cup each pineapple chunks, sliced strawberries, and grapes for fruit salad

1   cup low-fat fruit yogurt

6–8   whole-wheat crackers

Potato Bar Lunch

1	baked potato
¼	cup fat-free sour cream
½	cup shredded cheese
½	cup low-fat chili
1	cup apple sauce

Remind your child to reheat the potato and the chili in the cafeteria microwave for 2–3 minutes before piling on the remaining ingredients. She'll have as much fun making it as she does eating it.

Shapes Lunch

1	Low-fat tuna fish sandwich on whole-wheat bread, cut into triangles
½	cup round melon balls or sliced orange
½	cup oblong green grapes
½	cup cucumber slices, cut into squares
½	cup round sliced carrots
1	Rectangular low-fat granola bar

Your child will have fun seeing how many shapes he can find hidden in his lunch.

Chapter 11

Meals That Work

Rounding up your kids and shepherding them to the table for regular meals together is one of the best ways to teach them about proper eating habits and good nutrition. Although the foods that your kids eat are important, your presence at the table is critical.

Even when moms don't intentionally set out to make mealtimes educational affairs, kids learn a lot just by watching their maternal mentors. Mimicking their mothers' behavior, kids learn to exercise portion control, acquire proper table manners, and develop tastes for a variety of foods.

Set the Tone

Moms are in charge of setting the tone for each meal, which should emphasize relaxed dining and pleasant conversation. If you're the mother of young children, mealtimes will go a lot smoother if you have everything you need on the table before you sit down to eat. It's hard to enjoy your meal when you're jumping up every few minutes to retrieve forgotten items like bibs, sippy cups, and feeding spoons. If your kids are teenagers, try to navigate the conversation away from controversial and emotionally charged issues so that your dinner table doesn't become a war zone. Make sure that your kids know that mealtimes should be peaceful and pleasant for everyone present.

One of the most important steps you can take to promote positive interaction among family members is to turn off the television before you sit down at the table. Research has demonstrated that among families in which TV viewing is a normal part of the mealtime routine, diets include more pizzas, snack foods, and sodas and fewer fruits and vegetables than families in which eating and watching television are separate activities. In a recent study, researchers discovered that more than 42 percent of evening meals at home are consumed with the television on. The more frequently kids eat their meals in front of the television, the more likely they are to be overweight.

Try to keep the pace of your meals slow and relaxed and spend as much time in conversation as you spend eating. It takes about twenty minutes for your stomach to communicate the "I'm full" message to your brain for processing. It takes another moment or two for your brain to send a message to your hand that you've had enough to eat, and it's time to put the fork down. If you have a family of fast eaters who like to scarf down the entire meal in five minutes flat, they'll probably end up eating more than their bodies need. Before their brains get the signal that their stomachs are full, they'll probably be reaching for seconds. If your kids need help slowing down while they're eating, serve plenty of fiber-rich foods. Because they require more chewing, they take longer to eat than low-fiber foods. When your kids slow down the pace, they'll be able to focus more fully on the foods that they're eating. This higher level of awareness will help them eat less at each meal.

Keeping It Interesting

Children need a wide variety of nutritious foods for proper growth and development. To introduce your kids to different foods, try serving a new fruit, vegetable, or entree once or twice a week. Make sure to serve additional items that you know your kids will eat, just in case the new food is a total flop. Even if your kids won't eat it this time, don't throw in the towel prematurely. If it's a food that you enjoy, make it again for yourself and ask your children at least to taste it each time you serve it and keep any less than complimentary comments to themselves. Kids eventually learn to eat the foods that are put before them on a regular basis, especially when they see their parents eating and enjoying those foods. There's just no other way to explain the fact that children in other countries learn to eat and enjoy raw fish, the slimy internal organs of sheep and goats, and even creepy crawly insects.

Mommy's Little Helper

In addition to being a positive role model, one of the best ways you can motivate your kids to try a new food is to allow them to be involved in its preparation. Instead of shooing the kids out of the kitchen when it's time to fix supper, invite them to come in and join you. Kids love helping out in the kitchen. To a child, kneading real dough that will actually be made into bread or biscuits is a lot more exciting than playing make-believe with Play-Doh.

With a little instruction, kids can be handy little helpers. They can save you lots of time and energy by chopping vegetables, grating cheese, stirring batter, and mixing ingredients. Without a doubt, your kitchen will end up messier than if you prepared dinner by yourself, but the fun that you have talking and sharing is well worth the extra time it takes to clean up any minor messes.

Lessons for Life

When kids help out in the kitchen, they learn about more than just nutrition. They get fun, real-life lessons in math, science, and reading. Working as a team with siblings and parents to build their culinary creations, they'll be making warm memories that they'll cherish for a lifetime.

They'll also learn how to cook, a skill that has all but vanished among American youth. With very few moms making meals from scratch these days, many children grow up without ever learning their way around the kitchen. An entire generation of young Americans is incapable of preparing the most rudimentary of meals. Not only is this lack of skill a predictor of future poor health, it's also responsible for the loss of treasured family recipes and generations-old traditions.

As a mom, one of the greatest gifts you can give your child is the ability to fend for herself in the kitchen. When your child has the ability to prepare her own food, she has much more control over what she eats and, ultimately, over what she weighs.

Begin your children's cooking education with fun, simple projects that require only a few steps. As kids' skills increase and they become more familiar with cooking routines, recipes requiring more advanced abilities can be used. Teach children to use cooking utensils properly and safely. Whisks, measuring cups, strainers, and rolling pins are fun and easy to use and unlikely to cause dismemberment or other serious injury. As kids master the use of these tools, they can move on to more advanced technology, like graters, blenders, and ovens. Squeeze the most out of your cooking time by throwing in a few light lessons in math, science, and reading. Have your kids read instructions and nutrition labels out loud, pour and measure ingredients, and set the oven at the proper temperature. Teach your kids about the boiling point of water, the difference between liquids and solids, and the nutritional values of various foods. Even better, have your children amaze and delight you with their knowledge.

Designate one day of the week as cooking and baking day and have your kids join you for a few hours of fun in the kitchen. Have them help you prepare several meals at once so that you won't be tempted to stop by a fast food restaurant on your way home from work or be faced with the prospect of slaving over supper when you're already tired from a long day on the job. You can just pop a nutritious, premade dinner into the oven or onto the stove, steam some fresh vegetables, or throw together a salad. Not only will your family get better nutrition, you'll save yourself a lot of time in the long run.

On meal-making day, you can double your recipes or plan them for maximum efficiency. When you're browning ground beef for your chili, it makes sense to go ahead and prepare enough for a spaghetti dinner while you're at it. When you make seven or eight meals at once, your kitchen will stay cleaner throughout the week, and you'll end up spending less time washing dishes. The time that you save by not cooking each evening can be invested in fitness activities, like taking a half-hour walk around the block with your family or teaching your kids how to disco dance or do the limbo.

Do yourself a big favor and teach your kids one of the most valuable kitchen skills of all—cleaning up. Make sure your kids realize that cleaning up is just as important as meal preparation, and when it's time for kitchen duty, everyone pitches in.

Inviting your kids into the kitchen gives them an opportunity to develop valuable knowledge and skills that they'll put to good use for the rest of their lives. You'll also be giving them warm, wonderful memories that they'll cherish forever.

Time Savers

If you're a working mom, time is one of your most valuable assets. Don't feel guilty about taking shortcuts or using ready-to-eat ingredients whenever you can, as long as they're nutritious. To save time in preparation, you can buy fruits and vegetables from your supermarket's salad bar or nutritious side dishes from the deli department. Whole roasted chicken and precooked chicken strips can make meals a lot easier to prepare by saving you time and energy.

Quick cooking methods include indoor or outdoor grilling, stir-frying, and microwaving. Make good use of your time by adding extra items, like chicken breasts, to the grill. You can freeze them and reheat them in the microwave later for a quick meal with a great grilled flavor.

If you enjoy the flavor of marinated meats, take the meat out of its package when you get home from the grocery store and place it in a plastic freezer bag with your favorite marinade. Leave it in the refrigerator overnight and then freeze it for later use. Once it's defrosted, the meat will be full of delicious flavor, and all you'll need to do is fire up the grill.

Customize Your Recipes

Remember, recipes are nothing more than starting points. You can add ingredients or leave them out depending on what you have on hand and according to your family's preferences. If your kids hate garlic, leave it out.

If they'll eat green peppers but not mushrooms, don't hesitate to make the substitution. If a recipe calls for Colby cheese, and all you have is low-fat cheddar, don't let it stop you. Creativity and innovation are two of the most important skills you can bring to the kitchen.

Watch out for serving sizes. When your family of four eats a dish that is intended to serve six, don't forget to count the extra calories. If you want to help your kids and yourself exercise portion control, the easiest way to do it is to remove the extra servings before you dig in and save them for lunch on the following day.

When it comes to side dishes, it's hard to improve the nutritional value of fresh, whole foods. The time and energy involved in preparing delicious entrees is enough without having to worry about putting together fancy fruit and vegetable dishes. You can showcase your culinary skills and feature interesting or exotic flavors in your main dishes, but leave the side dishes to nature. It's hard enough to put a nutritious, tasty entree on the table without having to worry about fixing fancy fruit and vegetable recipes.

The recipes that follow are for main dishes. Whole foods, like fruits, vegetables, and grains, should be served as side dishes whenever possible. While it's easy to add lots of calories and fat to fruits and vegetables, it's hard to improve on the nutrition they offer naturally. Encourage your kids to eat lots of fresh fruits, steamed vegetables, and whole grain rice as side dishes. These foods are not only better for them, they're much easier for you to prepare.

Action Plan

✔ **Make good use of your Crock-Pot or a slow-cooker.** Save time and work in the kitchen by preparing the ingredients for your meal in the evening and just pouring them in the cooker the next morning before you leave for work. You'll come home to a great-smelling house and a tasty, no-fuss dinner.

✔ **Try to eat at least one meal a day with your children.** There's no better way to instill positive eating habits in kids than leading by example.

✔ **Serve a variety of nutritious foods.** Try to cover at least three of the five food groups at every meal.

✔ **Serve water with each meal.** Even if your kids drink a glass of fruit juice or milk, giving them a glass of water as well will help them meet their daily fluid requirements, improve their digestion, and avoid overeating.

✔ **Make mealtimes memorable.** Kids love special touches like dining by candlelight and drinking from fancy glasses.

✔ **Host an "international" night once a week.** Serve foods like tacos and burritos on Mexican night, pasta or pizza on Italian night, and stir-fry on Japanese night. If your kids have the time and interest, allow them to dress up or decorate the table accordingly.

✔ **Serve it buffet-style.** Save yourself a little work every now and then by serving buffet-style meals. Place nutritious ingredients in casserole dishes or mixing bowls and allow the kids to build their own potatoes, salads, or tacos.

✔ **Give someone else a turn.** Allow each of your kids to design and help prepare a nutritious meal one night of the week. Take a few minutes to go over their menus and discuss their choices. Ask them which food groups will be represented and whether the meal includes beneficial nutrients like calcium, iron, and fiber. Have them prepare a list of the ingredients they'll need and accompany you on the next shopping trip.

✔ **Write it down.** Have a pad of paper or a small chalkboard on hand in your kitchen and keep a running list of foods, ingredients, and other supplies you need to pick up on your next trip to the grocery store. You can also use it to keep track of kids' kitchen duty assignments or remind them what's good to eat in the fridge or cupboard for after-school snacks.

Ground Beef Stew

1	pound lean ground beef
6	medium potatoes, peeled and cubed
1	package (16 ounces) baby carrots
3	cups water
2	tablespoons dry onion soup mix
1	teaspoon Italian seasoning
1	teaspoon salt
1	10 ¾-ounce can condensed tomato soup, undiluted
1	6-ounce can Italian tomato paste

In a skillet, cook beef over medium heat until no longer pink; drain. In a slow-cooker, combine next six ingredients. Stir in beef; cover and cook on high for 4–5 hours. Stir in soup and tomato paste; cover and cook for 1 hour or until heated through.

Servings: 12   **Calories per serving:** 180
G-Factors per serving: Fat 4, Carbohydrate 26, Protein 10

Chicken-Broccoli Casserole

½	pound cooked chicken chunks
1	12-ounce package frozen chopped broccoli
½	cup fat-free sour cream
1	10½-ounce can reduced fat cream of mushroom soup
¼	cup grated low-fat cheddar cheese
½	cup crushed reduced-fat cheese crackers

Thaw frozen broccoli in microwave for 2–3 minutes; drain; set aside. Mix sour cream and mushroom soup in a large bowl. Add chicken chunks and broccoli; stir mixture well. Pour into casserole dish; cover with grated cheese; sprinkle crushed crackers on top. Bake uncovered at 350 degrees F for 25 minutes. Cover and allow to cool for 10 minutes.

Servings: 5   **Calories per serving:** 225
G-Factors per serving: Fat 6.5, Carbohydrate 19, Protein 22

Lightning-Fast Lasagna

12	lasagna noodles
¼	cup grated reduced-fat Parmesan cheese
3	cups fat-free cottage cheese
1	8-ounce package low-fat mozzarella cheese, shredded
½	pound lean ground beef
1	28-ounce jar reduced-fat spaghetti sauce with vegetable chunks
	Nonstick vegetable spray

Boil lasagna noodles according to package directions; drain; set aside. In medium saucepan, brown ground beef over medium heat until no longer pink. Drain off excess fat; blot with a paper towel. Pour beef into a mixing bowl; add spaghetti sauce; set aside. In a separate mixing bowl, combine Parmesan cheese and cottage cheese. Lightly coat a 9" x 13" x 2" baking pan with nonstick spray; arrange 4 lasagna noodles on bottom. Spread ½ cup of beef and spaghetti sauce mixture evenly over noodles. Spread ½ cup of cottage cheese mixture on top; sprinkle evenly with ½ cup Mozzarella cheese. Repeat process twice. Bake in preheated oven at 350 degrees F for 1 hour. Remove from oven; let cool for 15 minutes.

Servings: 12 **Calories per serving:** 281
G-Factors per serving: Fat 8.5, Carbohydrate 30, Protein 21

Sausage and Spirals

1	pound bulk Italian sausage
5	cups spiral pasta, cooked and drained
1	medium green pepper, chopped
1	28-ounce jar reduced-fat meatless spaghetti sauce
1½	cups shredded low-fat mozzarella cheese

In a skillet, cook sausage and green pepper over medium heat until meat is no longer pink; drain. Stir in pasta and spaghetti sauce; mix well. Transfer to a 13" x 9" x 2" baking dish. Cover and bake at 350 degrees F for 25 minutes. Uncover; sprinkle with cheese.

Servings: 10   **Calories per serving:** 248
G-Factors per serving: Fat 8, Carbohydrate 28, Protein 16

Broccoli Sausage Casserole

1	pound fully cooked Polish sausage, cut into ¼-inch slices
1	medium bunch broccoli, cut into florets
½	cup sliced red onion
1	14½-ounce can diced tomatoes, undrained
1	teaspoon sugar
3	cups cooked spiral pasta

In a large skillet, sauté sausage, broccoli, and onion for 5–6 minutes or until broccoli is tender. Add tomatoes and sugar. Cover and simmer for 10 minutes. Add pasta and heat through.

Servings: 13   **Calories per serving:** 186
G-Factors per serving: Fat 6, Carbohydrate 20, Protein 13

Easy Chicken Tenders

½   pound boneless, skinless chicken breast, cut into strips

½   cup whole-wheat flour

1   teaspoon poultry seasoning

1   oven browning bag

Pour flour into bowl; dip chicken strips into flour. Place in single layer in browning bag. Sprinkle with poultry seasoning. Bake at 375 degrees F for 30 minutes or until golden brown. Serve with ketchup, honey mustard, or barbecue sauce dip.

Servings: 5   **Calories per serving:** 188
G-Factors per serving: Fat 4, Carbohydrate 8, Protein 30

Super-Easy Spaghetti

12   ounces spaghetti

½   pound lean ground beef

1   26-ounce jar reduced-fat spaghetti sauce with vegetable chunks

Cook noodles according to package directions. In medium skillet, brown ground beef until no longer pink. Drain excess oil; blot with paper towel. Add spaghetti sauce to meat in saucepan; simmer for 10–15 minutes. Serve warm over noodles.

Servings: 6   **Calories per serving:** 362
G-Factors per serving: Fat 6, Carbohydrate 60, Protein 17

Zesty, Zippety Barbecue Chicken

6	4-ounce skinless, boneless chicken breast halves
1	cup barbecue sauce, any flavor
1	small onion, sliced
1	green pepper, sliced
1	oven browning bag

Pour barbecue sauce into small mixing bowl. Dip chicken in sauce, covering completely. Place in browning bag; top with onions and green peppers. Bake at 350 degrees F for 45 minutes.

Servings: 6   **Calories per serving:** 269
G-Factors per serving: Fat 5, Carbohydrate 21, Protein 35

Pineapple Chicken

6	4-ounce chicken breast halves
¾	cup fat-free Italian salad dressing
¾	cup unsweetened pineapple juice
¾	cup white grape juice

In a large Ziploc plastic bag, combine salad dressing, pineapple juice, and grape juice. Add chicken and seal bag; turn to coat. Refrigerate overnight. Pour contents of bag into casserole dish; bake at 375 degrees F for 35 to 40 minutes until tender. Serve with rice.

Servings: 6   **Calories per serving:** 131
G-Factors per serving: Fat 3, Carbohydrate 3, Protein 23

One-Skillet Barbecued Chicken

1	20-ounce can pineapple chunks, packed in juice
6	4-ounce boneless, skinless chicken breast halves
1	cup honey barbecue sauce
½	cup chopped green pepper
3	cups hot cooked rice
	Nonstick vegetable spray

Drain pineapple, saving juice. Set fruit and juice aside. Lightly coat a large skillet with vegetable spray and brown chicken on both sides over medium heat. Remove chicken and keep warm. In the same skillet, sauté green pepper and pineapple until pepper is tender and pineapple is golden brown. Stir in barbecue sauce and pineapple juice. Return chicken to the pan, cover, and simmer for 15 minutes or until chicken juices run clear. Serve over rice.

Servings: 6   **Calories per serving:** 381
G-Factors per serving: Fat 5, Carbohydrate 47, Protein 37

Turkey Time

1	6-ounce package cornbread stuffing mix
2½	cups cubed cooked turkey
2	cups frozen cut green beans, thawed
1	12-ounce jar reduced-fat turkey gravy
	Nonstick vegetable spray

Prepare stuffing mix according to package directions, omitting the butter or margarine. Transfer to a lightly coated 11" x 7" x 2" baking dish. Top with turkey, green beans, and gravy. Cover and bake at 350 degrees F for 30–35 minutes or until heated through.

Servings: 6   **Calories per serving:** 205
G-Factors per serving: Fat 5, Carbohydrate 28, Protein 12

Pork Chops in Tomato Sauce

4	bone-in trimmed pork loin chops (3 ounces each)
½	small onion, thinly sliced
1	8-ounce can tomato sauce
¼	cup chicken broth

In large nonstick skillet, sauté onion in butter until tender. Add pork chops; brown on both sides. In a small bowl, combine tomato sauce and broth; pour over chops. Bring to a boil. Reduce heat, cover and simmer for 10–15 minutes or until tender.

Servings: 4　　**Calories per serving:** 188
G-Factors per serving: Fat 8, Carbohydrate 6, Protein 23

Ham Tetrazzini

1	10¾-ounce can reduced-fat condensed cream of mushroom soup
1	cup sliced mushrooms
1	cup fully cooked lean ham cubes
½	cup fat-free evaporated milk
2	tablespoons water
1	8-ounce package spaghetti
½	cup Parmesan cheese

In a slow cooker, combine soup, mushrooms, ham, milk, and water. Cover and cook on low for 4 hours. Cook spaghetti according to package directions; drain. Add the spaghetti and cheese to slow cooker; toss to coat.

Servings: 6　　**Calories per serving:** 229
G-Factors per serving: Fat 5, Carbohydrate 32, Protein 14

Salmon Quesadillas

4   ounces fat-free cream cheese, softened

2   tablespoons fat-free sour cream

1   teaspoon dill weed

6   flour tortillas (7 inches)

4   ounces smoked salmon, flaked

2   cups grated reduced-fat cheddar cheese

In a small mixing bowl, combine cream cheese, sour cream, and dill. Spray one side of each tortilla with nonstick vegetable spray and place in skillet, sprayed side down. Spread with one-third of the cream cheese mixture; sprinkle with one-third of the salmon and one-third of the cheese and top with another tortilla, sprayed side up. Cook over low heat for 2–3 minutes or until golden brown. Turn and cook 2–3 minutes until cheese is melted. Repeat with rest of ingredients. Cut into wedges.

Servings: 6   **Calories per serving:** 265
G-Factors per serving: Fat 8.5, Carbohydrate 28, Protein 19

Sweet-N-Sour Chicken

1   pound cooked boneless, skinless chicken breast strips

1   medium onion, thinly sliced

1   medium green pepper, seeded and cut into thin strips

1   bottle sweet-and-sour barbecue sauce
    Nonstick vegetable spray

Spray large skillet with cooking spray; heat over medium heat until hot. Sauté onions and green peppers until tender, about 5 minutes. Add chicken and sweet-and-sour sauce; cook 2 minutes or until hot.

Servings: 4   **Calories per serving:** 229
G-Factors per serving: Carbohydrate Fat 5, Carbohydrate 12, Protein 34

Beef and Bean Soup

½	pound lean ground beef
1	small onion, chopped
1	16-ounce can diced tomatoes, undrained
2	cups sliced carrots
2	cups broccoli florets
1	15-ounce can Great Northern beans, drained

Cook beef and onions in large saucepan until beef is browned, about 10 minutes. Stir in remaining ingredients and heat to boiling. Reduce heat and simmer, covered, until vegetables are tender, about 10 minutes.

Servings: 4   **Calories per serving:** 257
G-Factors per serving: Fat 5, Carbohydrate 33, Protein 20

Oven-Fried Chicken

6	4-ounce boneless, skinless chicken breast halves
4	egg whites
¼	cup fat-free milk
¼	cup all-purpose flour
½	cup finely crushed corn flakes
1½	cups dry breadcrumbs

Beat egg whites and milk in shallow bowl until blended. Coat chicken breasts with flour; dip in egg mixture; coat generously with combined corn flakes and breadcrumbs. Spray baking pan with cooking spray. Place chicken in baking pan; spray generously with cooking spray. Bake at 350 degrees F until chicken is browned and juices run clear, 45–60 minutes.

Servings: 6   **Calories per serving:** 365
G-Factors per serving: Fat 5, Carbohydrate 36, Protein 44

Seasoned Chicken

6	4-ounce boneless, skinless chicken breast halves
1	envelope golden onion soup mix
1	cup water
3	cup sliced carrots
2	sliced potatoes
1	sliced green pepper
½	teaspoon seasoned salt

Place chicken in 13" x 9" x 2" baking pan; add carrots, potatoes, and green pepper to pan; arrange chicken and vegetables in an even layer. Mix seasoned salt, onion soup mix, and water; pour over chicken and vegetables. Bake at 350 degrees F for 55–60 minutes or until chicken is tender.

Servings: 6   Calories per serving: 257
G-Factors per serving: Fat 5, Carbohydrate 16, Protein 37

Creamy Chicken and Rice

4	4-ounce boneless, skinless chicken breast halves, cut into strips
1	cup reduced-fat cream of mushroom soup
½	cup of water
2	cups hot cooked brown rice
	Nonstick vegetable spray

Coat skillet with vegetable spray; cook chicken strips over medium heat until lightly browned. Pour in soup and water; simmer about 20 minutes over medium heat. While chicken is simmering, prepare 2 cups brown rice according to package directions. Serve chicken over rice.

Servings: 4   Calories per serving: 274
G-Factors per serving: Fat 6, Carbohydrate 18, Protein 37

Chicken Tomato Pizza

2   4-ounce boneless, skinless chicken breast halves, cooked

1   package pizza crust, 8–10"

6   ounces reduced-fat mozzarella cheese

1   14½-ounce can chunky tomatoes, drained

   Nonstick vegetable spray

Spread pizza dough into prepared pizza pan. Lightly spray top of dough with vegetable spray; sprinkle shredded cheese over dough surface. Distribute chicken and tomatoes evenly over cheese. Bake at 450 degrees F for 10 minutes. Reduce heat to 400 and bake for 5–10 minutes more or until pizza is lightly browned on top.

Servings: 4   **Calories per serving:** 376
G-Factors per serving: Fat 8, Carbohydrate 40, Protein 36

Southwestern Spaghetti

½   pound lean ground beef

2   cups water

1   28-ounce jar reduced-fat spaghetti sauce

1   8-ounce package thin spaghetti, broken into thirds

6   small zucchini (about 1 pound), cut into chunks

½   cup shredded reduced-fat cheddar cheese

In a large skillet, brown beef over medium heat; drain. Remove beef. In the same skillet, combine the water and spaghetti sauce; bring to boil. Boil for 6 minutes; add zucchini. Cook 4–5 minutes longer, stirring several times, or until spaghetti and zucchini are tender. Stir in beef; sprinkle with cheese.

Servings: 5   **Calories per serving:** 445
G-Factors per serving: Fat 9, Carbohydrate 70, Protein 21

Mom's Famous Fast Meatloaf

1   pound lean ground beef
1   10½ can 98% fat-free cream of mushroom soup
2   egg whites
1   6-ounce box herb flavor stuffing mix
    Nonstick vegetable spray

In mixing bowl, combine dry stuffing, egg whites, and cream of mushroom soup; mix. Add ground beef; mix thoroughly. Lightly coat 2-quart casserole dish with nonstick spray; add mixture and smooth with a fork. Bake at 375 degrees F for 30 minutes or until meat is fully cooked and top is lightly brown.

Servings: 6   **Calories per serving:** 239
G-Factors per serving: Fat 7, Carbohydrate 25, Protein 19

Sesame Ginger Chicken

½   bottle 3-ounce sesame ginger marinade
1   14-ounce package Oriental stir-fry frozen vegetables
1   pound boneless, skinless chicken breasts, cut into small strips
2   tablespoons water
    Nonstick vegetable spray

Lightly coat large skillet with nonstick spray. Place chicken strips in skillet; cook over medium heat until browned. Add frozen vegetables and water to skillet; simmer until vegetables are tender. Drain off excess water. Pour marinade over chicken and vegetables; simmer 3–5 minutes more. Serve over rice.

Servings: 6   **Calories per serving:** 230
G-Factors per serving: Fat 3.3, Carbohydrate 30, Protein 20

Salmon Cakes

2	pouches skinless boneless pink salmon
¼	cup fat-free sour cream
½	cup chopped red pepper
½	cup chopped onion
1	tablespoon lemon juice
½	teaspoon seasoned salt
2	egg whites
1	cup dry breadcrumbs

In mixing bowl, flake salmon; add egg whites and sour cream. Stir in chopped red pepper, onion, seasoned salt, and lemon juice. Add the breadcrumbs and mix to even consistency. Mold into patties, place in baking dish, and bake at 325 degrees F for 30 minutes.

Servings: 4   **Calories per serving:** 334
G-Factors per serving: Fat 5.5, Carbohydrate 50, Protein 21

Chili

½	pound lean ground beef, turkey, or chicken
1	12-ounce can dark kidney beans
1	12-ounce can light kidney beans
1	12-ounce can tomato sauce
1	2-ounce package chili seasoning mix
1	8-ounce can diced tomatoes

In a large saucepan, brown ground beef over medium heat until no longer pink; drain. Add remaining ingredients; simmer 1 hour over low heat.

Servings: 6   **Calories per serving:** 232
G-Factors per serving: Fat 4, Carbohydrate 32, Protein 17

Turkey Tortilla Rounds

4	7-inch flour tortillas
4	tablespoons fat-free cream cheese
4	slices reduced-fat smoked turkey
1	small cucumber, peeled and thinly sliced

Following package directions, warm tortillas to soften them slightly. Spread 1 tablespoon cream cheese on each tortilla. Top cream cheese with 1 slice smoked turkey; top with several slices cucumber. Roll each tortilla tightly; slice into 1-inch rounds.

Servings: 4   **Calories per serving:** 125
G-Factors per serving: Fat 5, Carbohydrate 9, Protein 11

Steak and Veggie Stir-Fry

¾	pound boneless beef sirloin steak, cubed
3	teaspoons canola oil
2	cups broccoli florets
2	cups cauliflower florets
2	cups sliced carrots
2	medium tomatoes, cut into wedges
1	tablespoon cornstarch
1	cup beef broth
1	tablespoon water
1½	teaspoons soy sauce
¼	teaspoon ground ginger

In a large skillet, stir-fry steak in 2 teaspoons of the oil until no longer pink. Remove and keep warm. In the same pan, heat the remaining oil; add broccoli, cauliflower, and carrots. Stir-fry until vegetables are crisp-tender. In a bowl, combine cornstarch, broth, water, soy sauce, and ginger until smooth. Return beef to pan; cover with cornstarch mixture. Bring to a boil; cook and stir for 2 minutes or until thickened. Add tomatoes; heat through.

Servings: 4   **Calories per serving:** 245
G-Factors per serving: Fat 9, Carbohydrate 18, Protein 23

Teriyaki Burgers

1	8-ounce can water chestnuts, drained and chopped
⅓	cup teriyaki sauce
2	tablespoons chopped green onions
1½	pounds lean ground beef
7	fat-free whole-wheat hamburger buns
2	medium tomatoes, sliced
	Lettuce leaves

In a large bowl, combine water chestnuts, teriyaki sauce, and green onions. Crumble raw beef over mixture and mix. Shape into 7½-inch-thick patties. Grill, covered, over medium heat for 6–8 minutes on each side or until beef is no longer pink. Serve on buns with tomato and lettuce.

Servings: 7   **Calories per serving:** 293
G-Factors per serving: Fat 9, Carbohydrate 28, Protein 25

Black Beans and Rice

1	15-ounce can black beans, undrained
¼	teaspoon lime juice
2	dashes cayenne pepper
1	14½-ounce can diced tomatoes
3	cups cooked brown rice
½	ripe avocado, cut into bite-size pieces
½	cup feta cheese

Place beans and their liquid in a small saucepan and stir in cayenne pepper and lime juice. Simmer over medium heat until heated through. In another small pan, warm tomatoes over medium heat until heated through. Put ¾ cup hot rice on each plate and top with one-fourth of the beans and one-fourth of the tomatoes. Sprinkle each serving with one-fourth of the avocado pieces and one-fourth of the cheese.

Servings: 4   **Calories per serving:** 379
G-Factors per serving: Fat 9, Carbohydrate 60, Protein 12

Quick and Easy Quesadillas

4   7-inch flour tortillas

1   12-ounce package precooked southwestern-style seasoned chicken
     strips or chunks

1   whole tomato, chopped

     1 cup chopped lettuce

½   cup chopped onions

1   cup salsa

1   cup grated low-fat cheddar cheese

1   cup fat-free sour cream

     Nonstick vegetable spray

Lightly coat skillet with vegetable spray; place on stove over medium heat.
Place one tortilla in skillet and spread 2 tablespoons of salsa on tortilla.
Sprinkle half of the chicken and half of the grated cheese evenly over salsa;
top with thin layer of chopped tomatoes, lettuce, and onions. Cover with a
second tortilla. Lightly brown bottom tortilla; flip and brown the opposite
side. Cut into wedges; serve with a dollop of sour cream.

Servings: 4   **Calories per serving:** 485
G-Factors per serving: Fat 10, Carbohydrate 56, Protein 41

Chapter 12

Energy Out

First, the bad news: The Surgeon General's Report on Physical Activity and Health recently lamented that American kids and adults aren't getting regular exercise. Nearly 40 percent of the nation's population seems satisfied to lead the totally sedentary lifestyle of a sofa spud, engaging in no form of exercise whatsoever. Another 40 percent of the population engage in physical activity haphazardly, meeting the criteria for "seldom" or "occasional" exercisers. Only about 20 percent of American kids and adults manage to squeeze regular workouts into their daily lives. If you and your children are not current and active members of the elite 20 percent club, it's time to get up and get moving.

Exercising regularly is especially hard for working moms. With a hectic schedule and a life that is full to the overflowing point, you may feel that you just don't have the time, the energy, or even the desire to work out. If you've hated exercising since you barely escaped sixth-grade gym class with your dignity, living the sedentary life of a garden slug may suit you just fine. But it's important to make exercise a priority in your life, if for no other reason than to set a good example for your children and to teach them the value of physical fitness. If you've been planning to exercise as soon as you can muster up the momentum or motivation, here's the good news you've been waiting for: exercising just got easier.

In the not too distant past, fitness experts led us to believe that in order for exercise to be beneficial, it had to be strenuous and continuous—at least thirty minutes a day, five days a week. If you weren't sweating, groaning, or having a near-death experience, you couldn't possibly be exercising effectively. Those who weren't able to put forth the effort dictated by the ivory-tower exercise purists simply resigned themselves to being the best couch anchors they could be. After years of doing nothing but watching TV and holding down the furniture, many of these folks fell so far out of shape that they couldn't exercise for thirty minutes if they sincerely wanted to.

But thanks to some intriguing new research, the rules regarding exercise have changed. Several studies have demonstrated that for people who are overweight, obese, or just plain out of shape, short, frequent bouts of activity are just as beneficial as longer, more intense exercise sessions. Results from the Physicians' Health Study, a project that has followed more than 22,000 U.S. male physicians since 1982, support this notion. Data from this study revealed that men whose daily exercise sessions lasted just eleven minutes had a 35 percent lower risk of suffering heart attacks than men who were total slugs. Surprisingly, exercising for longer periods of time didn't seem to lower the risk much more.

Men aren't the only ones who stand to benefit from brief, regular exercise sessions. In another study, researchers asked sedentary women to walk for twenty to forty minutes a day, either all at once or in ten-minute sessions. By the end of the study, both groups of women had achieved similar results in terms of weight loss and fitness gains. A similar study showed that women who walked ten minutes at a time, three times a day, lost at least as much weight as women who walked for thirty minutes at a stretch.

Based on these types of data, the American College of Sports Medicine recently adopted a new stance, recommending that formerly sedentary adults try to *accumulate* at least 120 minutes of moderate activity every week. Likewise, the latest federal guidelines recommend that American adults accumulate at least thirty minutes of moderate physical activity on most days of the week. Children and adolescents are advised to accumulate at least sixty minutes of moderate physical activity on most days of the week. The goal is to reduce the quarter-million deaths in the U.S. each year attributed to lack of regular physical activity—deaths caused by heart disease, cancer, and type II diabetes.

Even for time-strapped working moms, accumulating 120 minutes of activity over the course of a week is an entirely doable feat. If time pressures are great, you can get your 120 minutes a week by squeezing in several two- to five-minute sessions each day. You can grab a two-minute workout just by parking a little farther away from the grocery store, school, or office and hoofing it across the parking lot. You can pull all the dirty laundry off your treadmill and walk or jog the rubber road to nowhere for three to five minutes while your coffee is brewing in the morning. You can kick a soccer ball around the yard with your kids for five or ten minutes while dinner is cooking. The idea is to get your body moving—at any pace, for any length of time. If you can find just a few spare minutes here and there in your hectic day, you've got time to exercise. If you stick with it, the minutes and the benefits add up.

A Generation of Inactivity

Although it may seem that childhood is a carefree time of spontaneous activity and vigorous play, kids are becoming significantly less active with each generation. The lure of increasingly high-tech sedentary pursuits is largely to blame. Most kids today spend twice as much time vegged out in front of television sets or plugged into video games as they do exercising. According to the Surgeon General's Report on Physical Activity and Health, nearly half of U.S. youngsters between the ages of twelve and twenty-one aren't regularly active. Once children enter adolescence, exercise drops off dramatically, especially in girls. More often than not, this pattern of inactivity accompanies kids into adulthood.

Lack of regular exercise in childhood and adulthood contributes to a host of medical maladies, including heart disease, high blood pressure, diabetes, osteoporosis, and of course, obesity. These illnesses are currently the leading causes of disability and death in the United States, and they're expected to remain in the forefront well into the twenty-first century. Each year, an estimated 250,000 Americans lose their lives as a result of physical inactivity. For kids, lack of exercise not only reduces their quality of life—it practically sentences them to a lifetime of obesity, poor health, and premature death.

Unfortunately, American schools aren't providing a solution to the problem of inactivity in children. Just over a third of U.S. elementary and secondary schools offer daily phys ed classes. High school enrollment in gym class has declined in recent years, down from 42 percent of students in 1991 to just a quarter in 1995. Now more than ever, it's up to moms to promote exercise and activity in their children.

The Weight-Loss Equation

Remember the first law of thermodynamics from your old high school physics class? It still hasn't changed, and as it turns out, it applies to the human body as well as other entities. The first law of thermodynamics dictates that energy is neither created nor destroyed. As it applies to human beings, energy isn't created; it's consumed in the form of food. Nor is the energy destroyed; it is either released from the body through activity or exercise, or it is stored in the body for later use.

The human body expends energy in one of three ways: through the basal metabolic rate, through thermogenesis, or through physical activity. The basal metabolic rate is the minimum amount of energy expenditure required to carry on normal biologic functions and reactions in the body, such as breathing, keeping the heart beating, and carrying out the process of waste management. *Basal* metabolic rate is measured in a laboratory setting during complete and absolute rest, while *resting* metabolic rate can be measured at any time throughout the day. Energy expenditure during basal metabolic rate is about one calorie per minute, although it may increase slightly during the ingestion of food or with prolonged exposure to cold temperature. For the average sedentary person with a daily requirement of 2,300 calories, basal metabolic rate accounts for roughly 75 percent of the daily energy expenditure, or about 1,725 calories.

Dietary thermogenesis and physical activity are the other ways in which the body expends energy. Dietary thermogenesis is the energy expenditure required for the digestion, absorption, and transportation of food. Some individuals expend more calories in thermogenesis than others, and this phenomenon accounts for the slight metabolic differences between obese and lean individuals. In most people, dietary thermogenesis accounts for the energy expenditure of approximately 7 percent of the day's total, or 161 calories per day.

Physical activity deals with the energy expended during periods of exercise, and it accounts for around 18 percent of total energy expenditure, burning about 414 calories a day. While it was once thought that energy expenditure in the form of thermogenesis or basal metabolic rate was much lower in obese children than thin children, recent studies have disproved this notion. What *is* different is the number of calories expended through exercise. Low levels of physical activity are associated with higher levels of body fatness and an increased risk of obesity. In one study that examined the effects of an exercise program on kindergarten children, kids who participated in thirty-five minutes of exercise three times a week for five months were significantly less likely to be obese than those who were less active.

Data from the Framingham Children's Study examined physical activity levels over a five-day period twice yearly in a group of ninety-seven children from preschool through kindergarten. The inactive kids were nearly four times more likely to have higher percentages of body fat than those who were more active.

While there's not much you or your kids can do to change your basal metabolic rate or the number of calories you burn during the process of metabolizing your food, there's a lot you can change in the physical activity department. You can dramatically increase the number of calories you burn each day by increasing the frequency, level of intensity, or duration of the activities you engage in.

To maintain your body weight, the energy consumed in the form of food must be equal to your energy output each day. When these numbers are equal, there is an energy balance, and you neither gain weight nor lose it. In order to gain or lose weight, one or both sides of the energy equation must be adjusted. If weight loss is your goal, you must either reduce your energy intake or increase your energy output or both. If you decrease your daily food intake by 1,000 calories, or if you increase your energy expenditure by 1,000 calories each day, you'll create a negative energy balance of about 7,000 calories each week. Since each pound of body weight represents about 3,500 calories, a negative energy balance of 7,000 calories will result in the loss of about two pounds a week, which is the maximum amount recommended.

Another way to adjust the equation and still lose about two pounds a week is to decrease energy consumed in the form of food by 500 calories a day, while increasing the energy expended through physical activity to the tune of 500 calories a day. If losing two pounds a week doesn't sound all that earth-shattering to you, just remember that there are a total of fifty-two weeks in every year. Losing weight at a rate of two pounds a week, you could possibly drop around one hundred pounds in the next year, and that is *very* impressive.

The Lifelong Benefits of Physical Activity in Children

Though physical activity is most frequently associated with weight loss, exercise has so much more to offer—especially to the young. Exercise is a sound and largely risk-free investment in the current and future physical and emotional health status of children and adults.

Bone Development

Physical activity in kids has been shown to have positive, lasting effects on bone development. Exercise lowers the risk of developing osteoporosis by increasing bone mineral density. Although much attention is focused on exercise in middle and older age to reduce or restore bone loss, the human skeleton appears to be most responsive to the effects of physical activity in childhood, during periods of active growth.

Several studies have demonstrated that weight-bearing exercise performed three times a week for just eight months significantly increases density in the entire skeleton, particularly in the bones of the lumbar spine and legs. In fact, when regular exercisers were compared with nonexercisers, bone mineral density was found to be nearly double in the exercisers. Regular exercise before the onset of puberty appears to significantly reduce the risk of bone fractures early in life, and the protective effect extends well into adulthood.

Heart Health

While cardiovascular disease may not show up until adulthood, risk factors may begin to appear in childhood or adolescence. When they are present, they tend to persist and worsen throughout life. Research has strongly linked high cholesterol levels in youth with the development of high blood pressure and hardening of the arteries in adulthood, conditions that significantly increase the risk of heart disease and stroke. Kids who exercise show significant improvements in cholesterol levels and blood pressure levels. As a bonus, kids who engage in regular fitness activities are also less likely to resort to behaviors that are detrimental to cardiovascular health, such as drinking alcohol and smoking cigarettes.

Emotional Well-Being

In addition to promoting physical health, exercise has a profoundly beneficial effect on the emotional well-being of children and adults. People who exercise regularly have been shown to have lower rates of depression and anxiety and are able to cope with life's inevitable stressors more effectively than their sedentary counterparts. People who adhere to regular, rigorous exercise routines report less physical and emotional distress than those who spend more time in less strenuous pursuits. Kids and adults who engage in fitness-promoting activities enjoy improved levels of self-image and self-confidence and the happiness that comes with greater self-esteem.

Parents Shape Exercise Patterns

If you and your kids want to lose weight, keep it off, and stay healthy in the process, you absolutely, positively must exercise. Exercise is the primary predictor of whether or not you and your children will be overweight. If you're searching for a magic pill, potion, or gadget that will take the place of exercise, you're wasting your time and energy. In the time that it takes to procrastinate about exercising, you could have already finished a quick, effective workout.

Parents who live sedentary lives will find it difficult to motivate their kids to stay fit. A recent survey conducted by the National Youth Fitness Study found that home and community environments are the most important contributors to a child's fitness habits. Kids who watch more television, have less active parents, and don't participate in community activities tend to score poorly on tests measuring physical fitness.

The most important factor in the child-fitness equation is the support and involvement of at least one parent. The more moms get involved in their kids' fitness efforts, the more likely their children will be to remain physically active. You can promote fitness in your children by making exercise a part of your family's everyday life. It may take a little extra work to find fun fitness activities that the entire family can enjoy together, but your efforts will pay off for everyone.

Whether your kids are athletically gifted or not, they need your support in the activities they choose. Children who are encouraged to exercise in positive ways are likely to continue to enjoy exercise as they mature, so take care not to treat it as drudgery or a chore. Attempts to get your kids to exercise by bribing or browbeating them are also likely to backfire, as children who are forced to exercise in ways that they don't enjoy are significantly less likely to exercise as adults. Moms should give their kids a variety of choices of activities, sports, and physical education classes. Also, encourage your kids to come up with creative suggestions for family fitness activities. Kids who are involved in planning activities will be more likely to join in.

Exercising Through the Ages

If you want your kids to learn to enjoy exercise and remain safe while they're at it, it's important for you to help them choose activities that are appropriate for them. Factors to consider are age, interest, degree of physical conditioning, and stage of development.

Because no single sport or exercise regimen is best for children, it is far more important to find activities that each child finds interesting and enjoyable enough to stick with. Exercise for kids doesn't have to involve formal classes or rigid routines. As long as they're accumulating an hour each day of moderate activity on most days of the week, you can take comfort knowing that they're exercising enough to promote health, fitness, and emotional well-being.

Exercise for Infants

Because physical activity benefits the human body and brain at every age, kids should start exercising as babies. Infants need daily physical activity to help them explore and learn about their environments. Babies' activities shouldn't be restricted for too long, nor should they be confined to small play spaces or infant seats for extended periods of time. Movement should be fostered and encouraged early in life, and moms should make sure that their babies have plenty of room for creeping and crawling. If you're the mother of an infant, you can help get your child off to a good start by enrolling in a "Mommy and Me" type fitness program designed especially for moms and their infant children. If you're the do-it-yourself type, you can create your own program at home simply by getting down on the floor with your baby and encouraging her to move around.

Exercise for Toddlers and Preschoolers

As your baby matures into a toddler, you'll want to encourage her to get at least thirty minutes a day of adult-guided activity or play. At this age, it's not too difficult. Two- and three-year-old children live to play, and they thrive on unstructured activities like running, swinging, climbing, and water play. Chasing balls, playing tag, romping, and dancing serve the dual purposes of providing entertainment and exercise for children in this age group.

By the age of two, most children are able to jump, skip, and run. By age three, they've mastered changing directions from left to right and from forward to backward. Although they're gaining skills, toddlers still aren't quite mature enough to participate in organized sports or in competitive activities. While it's helpful to encourage your toddler to join in, don't force her if she doesn't want to engage in certain activities. You can always let her try again in a few weeks or months. For the time being, just move on to something else that she finds more interesting.

By the time your toddler becomes a preschooler, she'll be ready for up to an hour a day of active play. Moms should foster an active lifestyle by making sure that children in this age group are neither allowed nor required to sit still for more than an hour at a time. Preschoolers grow and develop rapidly, and they begin to master basic movements like jumping, kicking, throwing, and catching. They love to play active games with their parents and friends. As they learn to play in an increasingly coordinated manner, they may be ready to learn to ride bicycles, take karate lessons, or enroll in gymnastics classes. Some preschoolers are mature enough and sufficiently well developed to participate in organized sports, like swimming, T-ball, and soccer.

Because it can be difficult to keep small children interested and involved in sustained periods of exercise, moms have to be a little creative when it comes to designing fitness activities. When exercise or games take place in a group or a class setting, the size of the gathering should be small enough for each child to receive the individual attention, supervision, and coaching that she needs.

Exercise for School-Aged Children

Moms should continue to encourage their school-aged children to participate in unstructured, active outdoor play with their friends. From the ages of six to nine, children learn to refine the skills they learned when they were younger. At this point, sports participation and competition become a little more exciting. Although being the mother of a child athlete is a time-consuming and energy-zapping undertaking, it's important to encourage and support your child in the fitness-oriented activities she enjoys.

Kids between the ages of nine and thirteen can handle more advanced fitness endeavors. From a developmental perspective, well-developed teens can master just about any activity that they enjoy. Skateboarding, in-line skating, rock climbing, and snowboarding all qualify as great fitness activities. With kids in this age group, the major challenge facing most moms is keeping them interested in fitness and motivating them to stay active.

Remember to be patient with your child if she has difficulty finding an activity that she likes enough to stick with. It's not a good idea to force your child to take up activities just because you once excelled in them. Even if you were the high school cross-country champ, you may have to face the fact that your child doesn't share your zest for running—or the skill, for that matter. Many kids with superstar parents worry that they won't be able to measure up to the success that Mom or Dad once enjoyed in a particular sport and make a point of avoiding the very activities that their parents love. It may take a little time and experimentation before your child finds a sport, activity, or fitness hobby that she feels really passionate about, but your patience and encouragement will definitely pay off. Regular physical activity at every age will help your child learn a variety of skills that she'll need to meet life's challenges as she grows and matures.

Some kids may not be interested in participating in organized or team sports, but they can still keep fit by engaging in other activities that don't emphasize competition. As long as they don't slip into a sedentary lifestyle, there's no reason to worry or push if they resist joining organized sports activities. You can still encourage them to take up other activities like cycling, jogging, or martial arts. Not only do activities like these promote fitness in the short term, they also provide kids with fitness interests and hobbies that will probably last into adulthood.

Getting Started

No matter how motivated you and your kids are, if you're overweight or out of shape, you'll need to start out slowly, with just two to three sessions a week. Consistency, rather than intensity, is the most important skill to master initially. If an exercise program is started or progresses too abruptly, the likelihood of quitting is exponentially higher. Formerly sedentary kids and adults will progress at a much slower rate than their thinner, fitter counterparts and may have more muscle soreness and fatigue to contend with.

It may take a few months before you and your kids get into the rhythm of exercising. At first, it may even seem like work, but if you stick it out, you'll eventually begin to look forward to your workouts. Even in the early stages of an exercise program, you'll be rewarded with increasing stamina, flexibility, and strength. It won't be long before you start to see dramatic differences in your bodies.

(continued on page 232)

Target Heart Rate Zone for Moms and Teens

Younger children need to stay active, but it's not really necessary or even desirable to focus on increasing the intensity of their workouts. As they become more physically fit, they'll naturally step up their activity levels. Teens and adults, on the other hand, may want to work toward increasing the intensity of their exercise to make sure they're getting the most from the time they invest in fitness activities. Whatever type of aerobic activity you end up choosing, you'll probably want to increase the level of intensity by keeping your heart rate elevated for longer and longer periods of time. How high you strive to raise your heart rate depends primarily on your age. The average adult has a resting heart rate, or pulse, of about seventy to eighty beats per minute. As a general rule, the better your physical condition, the lower your resting heart rate.

The maximum attainable heart rate for most adults is about 220 beats per minute, and this rate declines steadily with age. It's not necessary—or even desirable—to elevate your heart rate to this point to achieve maximum cardiovascular benefits from exercise. For some folks, a heart rate of 220 beats per minute can be a little uncomfortable, and for others, it can be downright life threatening.

The target heart rate zone varies from person to person because it is a percentage of the maximum heart rate attainable for a person of a specific age. The first step in determining your own target heart rate zone is to simply subtract your age from 220. If you're forty years old, for example, you'll subtract 40 from 220, which equals 180. But don't worry; you don't have to get your heart beating to the tune of 180 beats per minute to get a good cardiovascular workout. You just need to step up your pulse to a number that falls between 70 to 90 percent of your maximum heart rate. The range of numbers that is 70 to 90 percent of your age-adjusted maximum heart rate is known as your target heart rate zone.

If you're forty years old, your age-adjusted maximum heart rate is 220 minus 40, or 180 beats per minute. Seventy percent of 180 equals 126, and

90 percent of 180 equals 162. If you're serious about getting the maximum cardiovascular benefit from the time you invest in exercise, you should exercise energetically enough to elevate your pulse to a point somewhere between 126 and 162 beats per minute and then keep it at this rate for at least twenty minutes. You'll need to repeat this process at least three times a week.

Before you go to the trouble of bumping up your heart rate, you might want to practice taking your pulse at rest a few times. You can usually feel a nice, strong pulsation at your carotid artery, the blood vessel that lies beside your windpipe in your neck about an inch or so below your jawbone. Be sure not to push on both sides of your neck at once, because you can cut off the blood flow to your brain, and you might pass out.

If you don't have any luck finding your carotid pulse, you might be able to pick up a good pulse at your radial artery. This blood vessel can be found on the thumb side of your inner wrist, just above the point at which your hand bone connects to your arm bone. If your radial pulse remains elusive, you may be able to feel the pulsation of your temporal artery, which lies just on the side of your forehead at your temple. Use the site that allows you to count the beats of your heart most easily.

If you located your pulse, congratulations! Now all you've got to do is count it. To count your heartbeats, press down lightly on the site you have chosen with your index and middle fingers. Using a watch with a second hand, count the number of pulsations you feel beneath your fingers for fifteen seconds and then multiply this number by four. This will give you the number of heartbeats per minute, or your heart rate.

It's important to determine your pulse by counting the beats of your heart for fifteen seconds and then multiplying by four, rather than counting for an entire sixty seconds. Why? Because as soon as you stop exercising to take your pulse, your heart rate drops dramatically, even in the first few seconds. The pulse that you count in the first fifteen seconds will most accurately reflect your true heart rate during exercise, and you'll want to give yourself full credit for your workout

Walking

It may help you to know that exercise doesn't have to be a "program." It doesn't have to be a complicated routine or ritual. It also doesn't have to be boring or painful or involve instruments of torture, like stair climbers, thigh-masters, or ab-doers. In fact, the more complicated you make exercise, the less likely you'll be to stick with it. You don't have to run six miles or pump iron for an hour a day to get a good workout. You just have to get your body in motion.

For kids and adults who are just starting out, exercising can be as simple as walking. In fact, walking is one of the most effective forms of aerobic exercise known to humankind. It requires no special training, and you and your kids don't have to be world-class athletes to do it.

For the new-to-exercise group, walking results in very few injuries. You won't end up sitting at home nursing pulled muscles or torn ligaments. Walking requires no special facilities or equipment. A good pair of walking shoes and some comfy clothes are all you and your kids need to get started. If you can find a quiet road, a park, or a shopping mall, you're ready to go. Best of all, walking is an incredibly effective form of exercise that the entire family can enjoy together. Walking elevates the heart rate, while it tones and shapes muscles. It burns calories, facilitates weight loss, and makes you feel great, both during the exercise and afterward.

You and your kids will get very real results if you walk at least three or four times a week. Walking at the snail's pace of just two miles an hour will burn up about 200 calories every sixty minutes. If you do this five days a week for an entire year, you can lose about fifteen pounds of body fat, without changing your eating habits at all.

Fitness experts recognize three levels of walking intensity. Strolling consists of walking a mile every twenty minutes. Although walking at this pace helps burn calories, it doesn't provide the same health benefits as more intense walking. You can do better than strolling.

Brisk walking is the recommended pace for most people. At a brisk walk, you'll cover a mile in about fifteen minutes, giving your heart and circulatory system a good workout. Depending on body weight, brisk walking burns anywhere from 250 to 400 calories an hour.

Fitness walking gives you the best aerobic workout, allowing you to cover a mile in about twelve minutes. Although the faster pace provides additional fitness and toning, it doesn't dramatically increase the overall health benefits you'll receive when compared with brisk walking.

Whatever speed you and your kids choose, walking will help each of you lose weight. For starters, walking removes you from the immediate vicinity of your kitchen. While you're out exercising, you can't graze a trail through the refrigerator or clean out the cookie jar. Walking also triggers the release of chemicals called endorphins, the body's natural appetite suppressants.

Walking increases muscle mass and reduces body fat. The more muscular your body is, the more calories it burns—even at rest. Walking increases the body's metabolic rate. For several hours after a thirty-minute walk, your body continues to burn calories at a faster rate than it would if you had stayed at home sitting on the couch.

When it comes to health benefits, walking does more than just promote weight loss. Walking just thirty minutes a day three times a week reduces the risk of developing heart disease by almost 50 percent. As an aerobic exercise, walking strengthens the heart. The heart is a muscle, just like biceps and quadriceps muscles. Muscles need regular exercise to stay in shape and grow stronger, and the heart is no exception. In kids and adults, walking lowers the chances of developing high cholesterol levels, high blood pressure, and type II diabetes. These illnesses are dangerous medical conditions in themselves, but they are also major contributors to heart disease.

Any type of weight-bearing exercise, including walking, reduces your risk of developing osteoporosis, a bone-thinning disease that can lead to fractures. The exercise also provides the stimulus that bones need to absorb calcium from food in the diet. As a bonus benefit for moms, exercise—including walking—can dramatically reduce the risk of developing breast cancer. A recent study published in the *New England Journal of Medicine* reported that women who exercise just four hours a week enjoy nearly a 40 percent reduction in the incidence of breast cancer as compared with more sedentary women. Whether you're trying to add years to your life or subtract inches from your waistline, walking is definitely a step in the right direction.

(continued on page 236)

Fluid Replacement During Exercise

Exercising kids and adults should take regular breaks to replace the fluid that is lost through sweating and respiration. Contrary to popular belief and commercially endorsed testimonials of name brand athletes, it *is* possible to exercise safely and effectively without consuming sports drinks.

The first of the popular sports drinks, Gatorade, made its debut more than thirty years ago when a few entrepreneurial types at the University of Florida came up with a million-dollar idea. They figured that if they analyzed the sweat of their Gator football players, they could design a drink that nearly equaled it to replace the body fluids and electrolytes lost during strenuous exercise. Because their concoction ended up tasting a lot like Gator sweat, they opted to disguise it with a hefty dose of sugar and some artificial coloring, and the rest is history. Gatorade and its wannabe competitors have built a multi-kazillion-dollar empire.

Sports drinks are supposed to ward off dehydration and fatigue by maximizing the body's absorption of fluid and high-energy carbohydrates during exercise. To be effective, the sugars in a sports drink should be primarily glucose, the fuel your muscles use for energy. If you're going to use sports drinks, look for ingredients like starch, maltodextrins, glucose polymers, and glucose—these ingredients provide 100 percent glucose. Although other sugars, like sucrose and high fructose corn syrup, taste a lot better, they aren't nearly as effective, as they provide only about 50 percent glucose.

The most popular sports drinks, Gatorade, Allsport, and Powerade, contain mostly fructose. Their relatively high sugar content causes them to be held in the stomach and actually pulls body water into the gastrointestinal tract, away from working muscles. Because they require more digestion, the body absorbs them more slowly than plain water, and the full stomach they create gives some exercising athletes a bellyache.

The salty taste you get with most sports drinks is just that—salt—made of sodium and potassium. These electrically charged minerals, called electrolytes, power working muscles, including the heart, during exercise. Sports drinks include sweat-mimicking proportions of electrolytes, but the truth is most folks lose insignificant amounts during regular exercise, and it's not really necessary to replace them right away.

In spite of all the sports drink hype, most people don't need them. Short workouts lasting less than an hour don't deplete the body of minerals or electrolytes. These deficiencies normally develop over longer periods of time, not after a jog around the block or a half-hour aerobics class. Realistically, you can get all the replacements you need from your next meal. After quick, intense bouts of exercise and sweating, you need only to replace your fluids, and plain old tap water will do the job just fine, thank you, and for pennies a serving.

If you and your kids are exercising to lose weight, sports drinks may not be the optimum beverage. The 150 or so calories that you worked so hard to rid yourself of can almost effortlessly and instantly be replaced by downing a 16-ounce bottle of your favorite sports drink.

If you or your kids exercise for more than an hour a day, congratulations. You deserve that sports drink, as well as a presidential award for physical fitness. You also need to take your fluid replacement very seriously to avoid dehydration. Endurance athletes can lose several liters of water and a substantial amount of electrolytes in the form of sweat.

If you're determined to drink a sports drink, you should be sure to follow the proper sports drink etiquette when you do it. For maximum effectiveness, the beverages should be consumed at a rate of 5 to 12 ounces every fifteen to twenty minutes during exercise. This rate of consumption provides a steady flow of fluids, energy, and electrolytes to ward off dehydration and fatigue. Sports drinks should always be served chilled, and the last swallow should be chased with a swig of water. Sports drinks are highly acidic, and when they're served warmed or sipped slowly, they're more likely to erode tooth enamel and promote cavities. Cold liquids are also absorbed more quickly from the stomach, speeding fluid replacement to working muscles and minimizing the discomfort that a full stomach can create during exercise.

Once you and your children have mastered walking and improved your level of fitness and endurance, you'll be ready to broaden your exercise horizons. You might want to move up to hiking, cycling, jogging, or swimming. For adventurous folks in search of a challenge, rock climbing, mountain biking, or in-line skating might fit the bill. As you and your kids become increasingly fit and gain self-confidence, your exercise options will continue to expand.

Resistance Training

With only about a fifth of Americans exercising on a regular basis, the surgeon general and like-minded health experts are diligently searching for new ways to get Americans up and moving. They recently gave their official and collective nod of approval to a type of exercise that many moms might find surprising—weight lifting. The American College of Sports Medicine and the American Heart Association give resistance training on enthusiastic thumbs-up for people of all ages and both genders.

While traditional belief holds that resistance training is dangerous for kids, it really isn't. It's endorsed by the Committee on Sports Medicine of the American Academy of Pediatrics as a way to improve fitness levels and increase strength, as long as kids are properly supervised and prescribed age-appropriate programs.

The safety and effectiveness of resistance-training programs for children, even prior to puberty, have been well documented. In addition to creating improvements in muscle strength, weight training benefits other aspects of fitness and performance, including flexibility and endurance. It bolsters cardiovascular health by lowering cholesterol levels and blood pressure and creates favorable changes in body composition, increasing the ratio of lean muscle mass to fat tissue.

By increasing bone mineral density, weight lifting reduces the risk of sustaining fractures and developing osteoporosis. It promotes fitness and conditioning and facilitates pain control in folks with arthritis and chronic back problems. It also enhances the health of people with diabetes by lowering blood sugar levels and boosting the body's production of insulin.

Weight training is often prescribed for children as a means of rehabilitating injuries, and it has been shown to actually help prevent some common types of sports injuries. Kids who engage in weight-training programs cut their risk of sustaining sports injuries in half. Strength training increases the strength and flexibility of muscles, tendons, and ligaments, decreasing the likelihood of sprains, strains, and tears.

The benefits of strength training don't stop with physical health. As they become stronger and meet the challenges of learning a new skill, athletes of all ages feel better about themselves. Greater levels of self-confidence and higher self-esteem are added benefits of weight-training programs.

Most kids can begin strength training as soon as they're developmentally and emotionally mature enough to participate in other sports. Even five- and six-year-olds can perform simple strength-training exercises like push-ups and sit-ups. Seven- and eight-year-olds can start working out with weights, as long as they can follow directions and use the appropriate amount of caution in the weight room. Even small weights can cause injuries if they're dropped on an unsuspecting foot or lifted improperly.

As with any sports or exercise program, it's important that your child visit her doctor for a physical examination before beginning a strength-training regime. Once your child has the doctor's thumbs-up, she's ready to go.

In the weight room, especially, moms need to make sure that children are properly supervised, using safe equipment, and following a routine that is appropriate for their age, strength, and level of development. Adult programs shouldn't be adapted for children. Not only are they too strenuous, they're also a little monotonous for kids with shorter attention spans. Weight-training programs for children should model the way kids play on a playground, with thirty- to sixty-second periods of activity interspersed with regular breaks.

While strength training is an excellent activity for kids and adults, there is an important distinction between weight training and weight lifting. The objective of a weight-training program is to improve total fitness, whereas weight lifting is a form of competition to see who can lift the most weight. Weight lifters, body builders, and power lifters train at high levels of intensity to become strong enough to move enormous amounts of weight. The focus of strength-training programs for kids should remain on increasing muscle strength rather than muscle mass, while exposing them to fun, safe, and effective training methods.

Bulking up shouldn't be the goal of a strength-training program for children. Younger kids and teens should work to tone their muscles rather than build them, combining low amounts of weight with several repetitions rather than lifting heavy loads just one or two times. Kids should never be allowed to perform single maximal lifts or sudden explosive movements. Weight lifting, bodybuilding, and power lifting should remain off limits until children's bodies are fully mature.

For people of all ages who are trying to slim down, pumping up can work wonders. Resistance training increases the percentage of muscle mass in the body. Pound for pound, muscle tissue burns nearly two to three times as many calories as fat. The more muscle mass you add to your body, the higher your metabolic rate, and the more calories you'll burn per hour, even while you're at rest.

One of the most attractive features of weight training is that even modest efforts can produce very real results. You and your kids don't have to hit the gym for hours every day to make major gains and realize dramatic differences in your bodies. While most traditional weight-lifting programs involve working out three days a week, even two days a week of resistance training is incredibly effective. In the first few months of an exercise program, lifting weights just twice weekly is nearly 90 percent as effective as working out three times a week.

When you and your kids pump iron a couple of times a week, it won't put a huge dent in your overcrowded schedule. It will also allow more time for muscle recuperation and dramatically increase the likelihood that you'll want to stick with the program.

For beginning weight lifters, resistance machines with adjustable weight stacks are generally recommended, since they're safer and easier to use than free weights. Resistance machines allow you to start with loads that are light in weight and work your way up to heavier loads in small, manageable increments.

Weight machines are designed to protect the lower back, reducing the likelihood that you and your kids will stress or strain the muscles of your back. While barbells and dumbbells require you to balance and control the weights on your own, resistance machines don't, so you'll be less likely to sustain an injury.

Working out with weight machines requires less time than free weight exercises, allowing you to complete your routine comfortably in thirty to forty-five minutes. Since exercise programs lasting longer than an hour have high injury and dropout rates, long workouts aren't recommended, especially when you're just getting started.

The key to success in weight lifting is to start low and go slow. When you can comfortably lift the weight that you're using for twelve repetitions with good form, it's time to advance to a slightly heavier weight. You should be able to increase the weight you're lifting by 5 percent at your next training session. On the other hand, if you can't lift the weight that you're using a minimum of eight times, the weight should be reduced at the next training session. Since level of effort and intensity are the critical factors in attaining maximum benefits, exercising to the point of mild fatigue yields best results. At this level of training, progression to a heavier weight should occur about every two to three weeks.

Whatever your level of fitness, weight lifting can be an important part of your exercise program. Whether you want to slim down or just shape up, resistance training could be your best bet.

Fitness for Life

No matter what sport or activity your child chooses, remember that fitness should always be fun. If your child doesn't seem to be enjoying herself, find out why and solve the problem if possible. If not, you can work with her to find another activity, one that she finds more appealing. Focusing on enjoyment and fitness rather than competition or winning is particularly important in organized sports. Kids who are pressured to compete or win may develop negative attitudes toward the sport itself and toward fitness in general. Make sure your words and actions reflect your belief that fitness should be fun. Try not to overwhelm your child with schedules that are jam-packed with sports practices and competitions or pressure them with unrealistic expectations. The reality is that most kids won't become Olympic champions or professional athletes no matter how much they practice, how hard they try, or how much you want them to succeed. The ultimate goal is to encourage children to become physically fit, healthy, and happy.

Action Plan

✔ **Make an exercise schedule.** Exercise doesn't have to involve a rigid routine, but it's a good idea to schedule a regular time for exercise each day. You and your kids will be more likely to get up and get moving if you've set aside a specific time for physical activity.

✔ **Plan your weekends and days off around fitness fun.** Plan a bike ride, take an invigorating hike along nature trails, or pack a picnic lunch and head for the park for a family game of Frisbee.

✔ **Make use of community resources.** When it comes to finding fitness opportunities, take advantage of what your community has to offer. Join the local YMCA or sign up for tennis lessons through your Parks and Recreation Department. Look for water aerobics classes and golf lessons at local swimming pools and golf courses.

✔ **Get the whole neighborhood involved.** Organize neighborhood fitness activities for children and their parents. Softball games, soccer matches, and jump rope contests are fun for kids and adults.

✔ **Dance!** Children of all ages love to dance. Crank up the music, show your kids the dances that were popular when you were a teen, and let them teach you their favorite dance moves.

✔ **Let your kids take turns being the fitness director for your family.** They'll have more fun when they're allowed to choose the activity, and they'll enjoy putting their parents and siblings through their paces.

Index

Entries in *italics* indicate recipes.